COME LIVE WITH ME TILL 90

and Beyond

Minoo Vazifdar

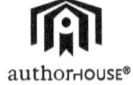

authorHOUSE®

AuthorHouse™ UK Ltd.
500 Avebury Boulevard
Central Milton Keynes, MK9 2BE
www.authorhouse.co.uk
Phone: 08001974150

© 2010 Minoo Vazifdar. All rights reserved.

No part of this book may be reproduced, stored in a retrieval system, or transmitted by any means without the written permission of the author.

First published by AuthorHouse 3/03/2011

ISBN: 978-1-4520-7418-4 (sc)
ISBN: 978-1-4520-7411-5 (e)

This book is printed on acid-free paper.

"The tragedy of old age is not that one is old
but that one is young."

Oscar Wilde

Author's note

This is a reality book. It is not written by an author who is 70 and conceptualises in his imagination what disciplines should be followed to achieve longevity. It is written by an author who describes his real life experiences for reaching the ripe old age 90 and now is in his 92nd year reasonably active, in good health with an enviable razor sharp memory.

I have expressed my strong belief in God, the power of prayers and divinity as they are the fundamentals on which human life is based and inward peace is realised. I have also taken the reader on a long dissertation of the need to have a highly compassionate view of the poor and needy and eradicate the destructive spectre of corruption because it takes away the resources meant for them.

Very recently scientists have discovered what they call the Methuselah (biblical patriarch who lived to 969 before the Flood and is considered to be the paragon of longevity) genes whose carriers have a good chance to be centenarians even with an unhealthy life style. It is made out that the right genes serve as a protection and is found in one person in 10000. I can not say what genes I have but my ancestors were not known for longevity and even my parents lived till the mid 60s only.

It is not my intention to denigrate India by writing that my longevity has been achieved in not an agreeable

environment which is largely true due to the pressure of the enormous population (1100 million) and the grinding poverty of the majority of people. This is why I have written fairly extensively in the Prologue a background to the evolvement of India until it became a united country and the difficulties it is facing. I love my country and I am a patriotic Indian.

Contents

Prologue

The Great Problem
On My Hand ----Is Vanishing
TIME

Living as I do, in state of instant mortality, at any time any place, I have been ruminating for some time now whether I should write down my thoughts for an enjoyable life to a very ripe old age for the benefit of tens of millions who despair on reaching their mid 60s as if their end is nigh.

Time is not batting for me. In my 92nd year I know I am living on multiple borrowed time. Before packing up for the night I thank the Almighty for giving me one more day on the planet with full possession of my limbs and mind and, before starting one more day of bountiful bonus, I pray that life will continue not with a burst but in its usual serene way. Bill Clinton, 42nd President of USA, on reaching 60, reportedly said that since now I have more

days behind me than ahead of me I try to wake up with a discipline of gratitude every day.

When I read the obituary columns describing the lives of successful people, with wide and varied accomplishments, dying in their prime and in their 60s and 70s I feel how fortunate I am to survive from practically the whole of the twentieth century to the next century today in 2010. However, the unexpected statistical factor announced its presence in early 2006 because may be I was looking too intently at my gift horse in the mouth. In January 2006 I was knocked down by a taxi resulting in fracture of the right ankle and other complications and I was out of commission for some time. After two months I resumed my normal activities with great resolution and strength of mind and put this unfortunate intervention out of my thoughts.

I am an Indian and my entire life has been spent in India which is not exactly a comfortable and easy country to live in if one is looking for longevity. It is a country of smells, noises and colours and one can easily add the all pervading dust. With the exception of colours, which are a welcome feature, the remaining three make an impact on one's quality of life and longevity. No matter what you do, noises, smells and dust follow you everywhere like your daylight shadow overwhelming you.

The street noise and unrestricted honking are deafening and continuous. The general low level of sanitary habits and inefficient conservancy services combine to provide a permanent malodour in the air and are the prime cause of

diseases. The clouds of dust in the atmosphere, caused by choking vehicular traffic with its uncontrolled emission and the teeming tens of thousands walking in the streets, with many shuffling their feet instead of lifting them, invade every nook and corner, stain clothes, stick on even perpendicular walls and leave a visible layer on your furniture requiring dusting twice a day. Imagine what quantity is inhaled to complete the picture.

Then there is the grinding poverty which smacks you in the eye. You cannot avoid it since 35% or nearly 400 million live below the line of poverty or subsistence level. The unfortunate poor sleep on pavements in tattered clothes, unwashed, unclean, doing menial jobs to earn some money to exist. I have, in a subsequent chapter, dealt with this subject extensively and its impact on mental equilibrium. There is a general feeling in India that this is the legacy of British rule of about 200 years, with little economic and social development, which left the country in a poor undeveloped state. This may be partially true but the problem is monumental and will take time to resolve.

Let me describe briefly the evolvement of what is called India which was not a homogenous one country. For approximately 200 years from 1526 it was ruled loosely by the Mogul emperors until the dynasty disintegrated. Thereafter, the country was torn by regional satraps and dominated by foreign trading companies of which the most prominent was the East India Company established by Royal Charter in UK in 1760. The trading companies

came to exploit the fabulous riches of the country. Alexander Dow in the History of Hindostan mentions India to be "one of the richest, most populous and best cultivated kingdom in the world". The consensus in 17th and 18th century was that India after China was the richest place on earth. To protect its trading interests, the East India Company's private army commanded by Lord Clive of India (he started as a clerk) gradually defeated local satraps and other continental powers, particularly the French, and established the hegemony of the Company over vast swathes of the country.

1857 was the watershed in the history of India when the rebellion of Indian sepoys (soldiers) was put down by a heavy hand. In history books this rebellion is dubbed as the Indian Mutiny but nationalist India calls it the War of Independence. It was notable for unspeakable brutality on both sides and the British are alleged to have fired live captives from the mouths of canons as a retribution to what their families suffered in the Mutiny. It was in this year that the East India Company was superseded and India as a unified country was brought under the British crown. This came to an end in 1947 on India becoming independent at the end of Second World War and Pakistan which was carved out of India became a sovereign country.

When the British consolidated India into one country and commenced their centralised active governance conditions, as compared to present times, were simply awful. Poverty, diseases, squalor, wretchedness and a very

inhospitable climate were thick on the ground and in the air. The rulers were prepared to face untold hardships, in a strange underdeveloped country, where the hot muggy period extended to eight months in the year. Diseases such as malaria, plague, diarrhoea, typhoid, cholera amongst others were the biggest killers and the life of an Englishman then was reckoned in the number of monsoons he could survive.

Unlike their predecessors belonging to East India Company who braved a hazardous 5 month voyage to Mumbai (Bombay) via the Cape of Good Hope before the Suez Canal was opened in about 1859 shortening the voyage to 21 days, young British civilians arriving via the Suez, after an apprentice period, were put in charge of large areas as District Collectors and Magistrates controlling and having absolute administrative power over 4000 sq. miles of territory inhabited by about one million people. Many times their posting was in remote parts of the country with not a single white soul to meet and talk to for miles.

This was the establishment of the Indian Civil Service (ICS) which came to be known as the heaven born "steel frame" of the British Empire in India-- incorruptible, competent, visionary, incapable of being dominated by politicians and they administered the districts with independence justly and fairly for the benefit and welfare of the poor people under their jurisdiction. This elite highly educated administrative corps numbered about 1000 both British and Indians.

With independence in 1947 all this markedly changed with the exodus of British members of the service and their replacement with competent Indians. The name was changed to the Indian Administrative Service (IAS) which became wholly Indian whose members were no less competent but circumstances made them succumb to political interference and domination with independence of action being chipped bit by bit until it is presently called the "bamboo frame". Now many work with one eye on pleasing their political masters to enhance their careers and one eye on their assignments.

In the very early days about 150 years ago they worked in primitive, inhospitable conditions in highly unsuitable climate at a time when there was no electricity, no transport except a buggy drawn by a single pony or horse moving at barely 10 mph or palanquin shouldered by human carriers. Riding the horse was the principal means of transport to administer the far flung areas of the district. They lived in uncomfortable bungalows (ground level structure with spacious garden) where drainage had to be covered by metal trellis to prevent snakes from venturing in and wild animals roared in the silent beautiful starry nights (India then boasted of may be 50,000 tigers as compared to barely 1500 now). In the summer months (April to June), to get some relief from the scorching heat and humidity, a man was employed to fan the "sahib" as he was respectfully called. Very few married and remaining single was actually encouraged. The British cadre intently

looked forward to the perk of 3 months leave after every 3 years of service when most of them went to UK.

There was hardly any social intercourse between the British rulers and Indians, with the latter expected to close their umbrellas and dismount if they were riding a horse in the presence of a white man. The maximum penalty for the British convicted of murder was a fine of Rs.150 (about $30 then). Lord Curzon, the British Viceroy, noted in his diary in 1901, that no European was convicted whatsoever the evidence. This was a part of the privilege of the ruler and it must be said that the British never ran amuck as some of the continental powers did in dark Africa.

The British built an Empire of which India was the Jewel in the Crown with a population of 400 million in undivided India in 1947, which included Pakistan, and governed by an elite administrative corps of civilians. It is unbelievable that this vast country with an enormous population was controlled by 60,000 troops of whom only 10,000 were British. They may have exploited the country economically but their achievements as colonisers were not inconsiderable.

They enacted laws which have survived till today with few amendments. They set up a vast railway system extending to about 54,000 km (36,000 miles) interconnecting and unifying a huge country enabling easy movement of people and food grains to protect against famines and developing trade and commerce. This was all at a time when there was hardly any mechanical

construction equipment available to lay down tracks and build thousands of bridges. The British railway rolling stock industry was booming supplying to India.

They developed trade and commerce albeit to enrich themselves, built ports, established postal and telegraph systems, universities and municipalities, a dependable medical health care organisation, regulations for protecting India's monuments and temples and established the rule of law with a civil and criminal code which to this day remains largely unchanged.

They spread the English language which, for generations of Indians in urban areas, has been a window to the world of education, technology, scientific advancement and for establishing the foundation of democracy. Proficiency in English of the Indian urban educated class has been the driving force for the accelerated economic development of India with an annual growth rate which is the highest next to China.

Nevertheless the greatest blot in the history of British rule was their surprise and sudden decision to leave India in August 1947 without putting in place effective control in the midst of burning fires of deep distrust and disagreement between Hindus and Muslims caused by the Partition of India due to carving of Pakistan. This led to the mass migration of hundreds of thousands of Hindus from Pakistan and vice versa of Muslims from India to Pakistan with killings and uncontrollable atrocities resulting it is estimated in nearly one million deaths.

Despite all efforts when the British left in 1947, one out of five newly born died before attaining the age of one and life expectancy hovered at about 35. Since then there has been a measurable improvement with emphasis on health care and medical facilities, better sanitation, improved environment, education and the endeavour of the people themselves wanting to enjoy a better life style. However, this turn of affairs has led to the unfortunate consequence of population increasing from 320 millions in 1947 for divided India (excluding Pakistan) to about 1100 millions today. The reason is that though there has been some increase in the number of people born, less and less people are now dying. Consequently, the enormous economic development of India has little to demonstrate, except in the urban areas, with the national per capita income at an abysmal low figure of about $ 800/1000 per annum.

In large parts of India, particularly in villages which number about 550,000, and where real India lives, due to increase in population, medical care and health facilities even at an elementary level are stretched to the limit. Sanitation continues to be the minimum being barely a hole in the ground in the majority of villages. In rural areas, it is usual to venture out early in the mornings for ablutions which, when wild life was stalking the countryside, was highly risky and disastrous. According to the report of the Development Committee of the IMF and the World Bank, the South Asian region is worse off than the sub-Sahara regions with 35 % only having

access to improved sanitation facilities. In India 60% or 660 million people do not have piped, clean unpolluted drinking water and deaths due to water borne diseases are at the highest level.

Is it believable that the manifesto of a leading political party for the 2007 Mumbai (Bombay) municipal elections, with a population of 14 millions, brazenly speaks of providing supply of adequate unpolluted water and the cleaning of sewage and gutters and this is 60 years after self- rule!!

Electricity has reached only 40% or 440 millions with tens of millions having just a single incandescent bulb to illuminate their lives which also is subject to horrendous power cuts and sudden shortages particularly in the hot and humid summer months. Only 200,000 villages or 36 % are electrified. In the large northern belt of India, where about 35% of population or 400 millions live, households without electricity range from 70 to 80% and they have to make do with kerosene lanterns. It has been remarked, with a large element of truth, that having nothing to do the parents retire early and procreate and if they were provided with dependable electric power they would read or enjoy television instead, providing another way of birth control.

Health and medical care are still at an abysmal low level. India accounts for 33% of the world's diarrhoeal diseases and 25% of maternal deaths. There is inadequate institutional social security to take care of the aged and the

infirm and when they retire, they return to their villages to pass the rest of their lives in peace and die.

There are millions of people living in India's cities. About 14 million live in the city of Mumbai and the impact of people, more people and still more people is everywhere. In every city there are unbelievable crowds on the roads and pavements. They push, jostle and elbow you out of the way as every one is in a tearing frenetic hurry and the words "sorry" or "excuse me" are totally unknown and a physically challenged person should not expect any special courtesy when walking.

Urban transport, be it suburban trains or buses, is groaning under the weight of unimaginable crowding. People have to fight to get into suburban and long distance trains and fight to get out. On suburban lines, they hang by the proverbial thread clutching to whatever is nearest, sometimes losing their balance and dying a horrible death on the tracks. Those who can not get even any tiny space, climb on to the top and get electrocuted. Roads are clogged with cars, vintage taxis and heavy vehicles plying with inadequate regulatory control, road discipline and etiquette endangering lives. Drivers generally are on a dare devil mission cutting in and out on the left and right.

The urban centres are a mass of architecturally painful concrete jungles with little development planning and breathing space. New buildings coming up as replacement for shanty towns are shoddy poorly constructed and are unlikely to last even for 20 years. Cities are left gasping for fresh air. In Mumbai open space is 0.03 acre per 1000

people (Greater London and New York have 12 and 4 acres respectively).

Presently, it would be no exaggeration to say that what one eats has to be sanitised, what one drinks has to be boiled and filtered and on top of this breathe the polluted air. In all this environment, if I have survived going into age 92, with mental acuity, physical bounce, thirst for peaceful life and its pleasures should be a signal to all those who, when they turn 60/65, despair of ageing and the life to come accepting gradual disintegration into old age. To them and they run into tens of millions I would send the message that life is for living and not for moaning. One must not let life's dusk stage to relapse into darkness. To make this possible is all in one's hands to follow certain painless disciplines and create the necessary environment so that thistles and not prickles are gathered. In life things don't happen you have to make them happen by positive attitude, self-efforts and discipline.

I am bold enough to say that I am the living example of credibility to write this book and unfold my plan to live and enjoy life up to 90 and beyond. At my age I have had the energy and motivation to write, using my prodigious memory to remember various events, marshal facts and review and screen what I have read to present in book form working on a lap top without a secretary or assistance from a ghost writer?

TIME magazine, in its October 17 2005 issue quoted the following excerpts from Andrew Weil's book *Healthy Ageing:*

"I recently turned 60. To help celebrate the occasion, friends organised a surprise party. After the festivities, there came a time to reflect, and I came to an uncomfortable conclusion. I am closer to that period in life when my energy and powers will diminish and I will lose my independence. At age 60, the organs of the body gradually begin to fail and the first hints of age related diseases begin to appear. I hardly notice my aging on a day to day basis. When I look into the mirror each morning, my face and white beard seem the same as the day before. But in photographs from the 1970s, my beard is completely black. On closer inspection, I notice other changes in my body-- more aches and pains, less resilience, less vigour. And my memory may not be quite what it used to be. At the same time, despite the evidence, some part of me feels unchanged."

I have not read the book but the excerpts are interesting and I was then 25 years older to him.

Let me introduce myself to the reader. I am 1.70m tall and my weight has been constant for the past 50 years at about 70 kilograms with a BMI (Body Mass Index) of about 24. In the past 40 years I have been treated for injuries arising from a car accident, removal of hernia and cataracts. I walk a lot both as an exercise and at home and used to play a round of golf twice a week. I may be suffering from a few inconsequential infirmities but they are par for a man of my age. After the car accident in 2006 at age 86 I have become somewhat unbalanced in

my walk and for protection carry a stick and regrettably because of lack of balance I am unable to play golf.

I was educated in Mumbai obtaining a Master's degree in Commerce and Economics and was later seconded for a 12 weeks course in higher management at the Administrative Staff College, Henley-on-Thames, UK.

I was a senior executive in India's largest business and industrial conglomerate the TATA Group and was the Managing Director of a mid-sized company. Later, I was associated with a chamber of commerce and industry dealing with France and for my work the French Government in 1988 conferred on me the title of Chevalier de L'Ordre National du Merite.

I go to sleep at midnight and sleep for 7 hours accompanied by a half hour afternoon siesta which is a must for me to be physically active and mentally alert till midnight. The latest study, however, advises that 10 hour sleep is the key to live till 100 as it is a major factor in rejuvenating the body, activating the immune system, regenerating human cells and removing toxins.

I have a good appetite but my quantitative intake is strictly controlled. I do not follow any structured diet but impose on myself strict quantity restriction, which I have described in detail, as one of the most important disciplines to follow. I do not drink alcohol as a habit and indulge in an occasional glass of beer and a peg of Scotch as social conviviality at rare parties or functions. Sometimes I do drink a half glass of red wine with dinner and occasionally a peg of brandy.

I am fond of playing bridge. I read a lot and avoid all types of light reading matter. I do simple calculations by memory which keeps my mind sharp and alert and can relate international and national events going backwards to 70 years ago to the commencement of the Second World War.

With advancing age, if mental faculty is all there, the only physical experience of ageing will be some creaking of bones and instability in movements but all the normal actions like driving a car, walking, travelling, performing household chores, having a reasonably healthy appetite and mild sexual activity are all within range. I feel very encouraged that at my age I travel alone for pleasure once a year and in past 3 years I have visited Washington, New York, London and Paris walking for miles to enjoy the delights of the places visited.

In this narrative no attempt is made to push death away which should be accepted, as the ancient Egyptians did, as simply the beginning of a journey to another world. I am not a martinet striving for difficult, if not impossible, standards. I believe that to achieve longevity the disciplines I have emphasised are easily within reach accompanied by mental alertness, the right attitude and always positive focus. The whole exercise is to ensure that, as one advances in age, there is fulfilment to be enjoyed and I am writing based on personal experiences of one who reached 60 in 1979 and is now in his 92nd year.

It may appear that I have dealt at length in this book with the subjects of faith, belief in God and religion and

the existence and eradication of poverty in the quest for promoting a long life span but this is not so. In fact, there is much to write on these subjects but I felt, if I did, I would be drifting away from the main message of this book. I honestly believe that mental peace and equilibrium for a long, purposeful, healthy life can only be realised if you believe in the existence of God and are mindful of and care for the poor and the disadvantaged to bring light in their lives. As Orphan Pamuk said when receiving the Nobel Prize in Literature at Stockholm in 2006 "The frustrations, hostility and anger generated by abject poverty cannot sustain peace in any society in the world". Also, every one in India should take corruption head on as it is so endemic in every walk of life that it could be classified as a moral meltdown since it takes away a part of the relief resources meant for the poor.

In writing this book I have tried to be as brief as possible bearing in mind Shakespeare's aphorism "Brevity is the soul of wit". To be a part of two centuries, a full 81 years of the 20th and now in the 21st is a great joy. I commend to the reader that the views I have expressed if followed would have a strong lasting effect on his life span.

Chapter I

**"If we pray we will believe
If we believe we will love
If we love we will serve."
Mother Teresa**

God and Religion
Great Importance to Longevity

The abiding influence in my life, which I firmly believe has led to my long life span, is my belief in the existence of God, the Hand which guides humanity. Whether one accepts this assertion or not is a matter of individual choice. In my view those who do, enjoy both temporal and spiritual contentment and those who do not are living may be in a state of denial.

God cannot be expressed in the human form to be touched and worshipped. If God is human he would be instantly mortal. Those who believe reach Him through various paths ultimately leading to one God. The great religions Christianity, Islam, Buddhism, Judaism,

Zoroastrianism and Hinduism which is a collection of philosophies, are all giant steps to divinity.

Hinduism is a way of life and does not involve the exclusive worship of a single god, sage or prophet and has no book of prayers like the Bible, Koran or Torah. The Vedas which are a collection of hymns and chants are the earliest sacred texts of Hinduism. Then came the philosophical Upanishads followed by the great epics the Ramayana and the Mahabharata which, through stories and fables, deal with the inner conflict between the human soul and senses. Christianity, Islam, Judaism and Zoroastrianism are monotheistic religions enjoining on their followers the worship of one transcendent God only. Budhism is the most tolerant marked by non-violence and devoid of any dogma. In Budhism individuals do not have a God to worship but strive to seek enlightenment or Budhahood through meditation. Three essentials to Budhism are do no harm, perform right actions and meditation by training the mind.

Polytheistic Hinduism is very liberal and epitomises with its large Hindu believers the secular nature of India by respecting and tolerating all faiths. Now with the caste barriers broken anyone can walk into a Hindu temple. The finest example is having a Muslim pujari (priest) reciting prayers in Sanskrit and performing all the normal rituals and blessing devotees at a Durga temple in an obscure village near Visahkapatnam in north east India. A Hindu can worship at any non - Hindu shrine without affecting his status as a Hindu. In Mumbai, Hindus

participate in Christian festivals and also visit Muslim *darghas* (shrines or tombs of holy men). The late Bismillah Khan, a Shia Muslim, who was India's greatest Shenai musician, worshipped Saraswati, the Hindu goddess of music, and his uncle was the official Shenai player at Varanasi's (Benaras) famous Hindu Vishwanath temple.

As I am a Zoroastrian a few words about my religion, which is relatively unknown, may not be out of place for the reader. We worship Zoroaster (628 BC) as the prophet and the founder of the religion which professes the monotheistic concept of God. Religious historians have speculated on connection between Zoroaster's teachings and Judaism and Christianity and some have even extended it to Islam. According to historians, Zoroaster flourished 260 years before Alexander the Great. Whilst Zoroaster is our prophet, our God is Ahura Mazda (Ohrmazd), the Wise Lord, the Creator of Heaven and Earth, the spiritual and material worlds. Our scriptures are the Avesta and our hymns are called the Gathas.

The principal element of our worship is the fire which is kept ignited with sandal wood when we pray. A distinguishing feature of our religious practice is we do not bury or cremate our dead but leave them in a circular enclosure called the Towers of Silence for vultures to feed on and now since there are no vultures in large urban areas, the bodies are putrefied by directing the sun's rays on them. I believe the Chinese Tibetans have much the same system except that they chop up the corpse and leave it on top of the hill.

The distinguishing face of Zoroastrians are the Parsis of India. About 80 fled Iran 1300 years ago in sail boats to avoid persecution and forced conversion to Islam and landed on the shores of western India and were given refuge by the then reigning Hindu King. The community is tightly knit, is largely prosperous through trade, commerce and industry and is known for handsome charities and shuns proselytization. The number which grew to more than 100,000 in India, mainly in Mumbai, has now dwindled to 60,000 with many migrating to UK, Canada and USA. As conversion is not allowed our future is dim but it is believed there are several thousand Zoroastrians (not Parsis) in the Caucasian countries and some also converted, not acceptable to orthodoxy, in California. To stem the dwindling population which, if not controlled, will lead to extinction and Parsis will then be known as the lost tribe of India, measures are taken to encourage growth by offering families a maintenance allowance of $75 per month each for second and third child until they reach age 18.

All religions lead to the Supreme God, the Creator of life and the Provider of natural means to sustain life. There is no conflict or divergence between the religions in their eternal search being complementary to one another. I am not a religious scholar but I understand Jesus is mentioned 17 times in the Koran and special reference is also made to Abraham? During his visit to a very rare functioning Christian church on a state visit to China in November 2005, Mr. George W. Bush, the former President of USA

said, what is very true, that a healthy society is a society that welcomes all faiths and gives people a chance to express themselves through worship of the Almighty.

After centuries of hostility and bitterness Pope Benedict XV1 showed his eagerness to mend fences by inviting the President of Israel to visit the Vatican to mark a new era of reconciliation between Christianity with 1600 million and Judaism with 14 million believers. This historic event was the first such visit in 2000 years and is a part of the Vatican's inaugural pledge to reach out to other faiths. Recently, the Pope on his visit to Turkey not only expressed in favour of Turkey joining the European Union but, when visiting the magnificent Blue Mosque, His Holiness turned towards Mecca and prayed which symbolic gesture appeared to have gone down well with his hosts. But what is extraordinary and significant is that following the visit of King Abdullah of Saudi Arabia to the Vatican, the first Roman Catholic Church is likely to be established in the Islamic Kingdom where church worship is banned and it is an offence even to possess a rosary, bible or crucifix.

Islam, which is a great religion worshipped fervently by 1500 million people (one in every four on the planet) is stretching the hand to all those, who never cease to revile it, by allowing the establishment of the first Christian church, since its arrival in the 7th century, at Doha in the Islamic state of Qatar. As the Most Reverend Clive Handford, the Anglican bishop of Cyprus said "We hope that the centre can be a base for ongoing Muslim-

Christian dialogue". Some pro western Gulf states have indeed allowed Christian churches, wherever there is a sizable Christian population, but Qatar is quite special as it is the home of *AL –JAZEERA*, the Arab news network, which became famous with the reporting of the Iraq war and periodic bulletins issued by Al-Qaeda.

No matter what religion is worshipped they are all esoteric, full of content, commanding respect and deliver to the worshipper a great feeling of composure and mental peace. In Christian churches, the hymns, choirs, organ recitals, mass, requiems of Handel, Bach, Beethoven are divine and arouse spiritual, inspirational and emotional uplift leading to peace and contentment.

There is revival of religion in China and religion appears to be taking big strides again in large parts of Russia, after Marx, Lenin and Mao Tse- tung had the most destructive impact on worship in the two countries in the last century exterminating the deep seated teachings of Christ, Buddha, Tao and Confucius leaving millions without any spiritual support and sustenance in the dark times of very harsh communist regimes and destructive wars.

Already, after the fall of communism, there is a revival of religious worship in Russia and Mongolia. When Russia mocked religion, churches were converted into museums of atheism, the most notable being St. Peters but delightfully St. Peters is back as a cathedral. The Russian Orthodox Church with the personal recognition and encouragement of Prime Minister Vladimir Putin is

having a significant revival particularly amongst the youth of the country, which is refreshing, as compared to what I saw on my two visits to Moscow in the late 60s when the only worshippers were the old and a sprinkling of young girls who were probably escorting their mothers and grandmothers. Even in China, where religious worship is taboo, there is a revival, fuelled by liberation caused by the economic boom, but unfortunately the worship is still very clandestine as the state frowns upon religion.

God's generosity, compassion, protection and creativity are attributes which make life and living possible. However, His Kingdom is assailed today by doubts and interrogation. Questions asked are if He is compassionate, merciful and relieves distress why is there so much suffering and inequality in the world? Why is mankind visited with calamities like earthquakes, hurricanes, tidal waves, typhoons which leave in their trail vast destruction of life and property causing unbelievable misery to humanity? Is Alexander Dumas right in saying "If God is condemned to live the life he has inflicted on others, he would kill himself".

Tsunami hit Asia in last week of December 2004 claiming 300,000 lives leaving enormous destruction affecting the livelihood of a million people. Hurricane Katrina struck New Orleans with terrible ferocity destroying the whole city with horrific death toll. The entire city of 250,000 would have to be rebuilt, before the population could be allowed to resettle, at an astronomical cost. This was followed by hurricanes Rita

and Wilma. In October 2005, a devastating earthquake in Pakistan killed 73,000 and rendered nearly 3 million homeless. 2010 began with a vastly destructive 7 Richter scale earthquake striking poverty stricken Port-au-Prince causing deaths and destruction on an unimaginable scale. These are not just isolated calamities. 60,000 people died in Lisbon in1775 due to a devastating Tsunami, following a subterranean earthquake.

Also it would not be wrong to question why is there such a deep gulf between the rich and the poor, the latter forming a far larger proportion of human beings on the planet? Why does God, if he is merciful and beneficent, allow poverty and destitution stalk a large part of the world particularly in Asia and Africa? One can relate many similar questions to doubt the existence of God. It has not been possible to dismiss these eternal doubts by logic and analytical probing. Over the ages, great minds and thinkers have endeavoured to do just that without satisfaction. This lack of acceptable explanation is merciful because otherwise God would be subjected to scrutiny and response and what we know as the fact of the Unknown, which is the foundation of our belief, would be fatally pierced.

A question was asked 50 years ago "Should God dwell in hell" and Dr. Savepally Radhakrishnan, Professor of Eastern Religions and Ethics at Oxford University (1936-52), renowned philosopher who ultimately became the President of India, at a meeting organised by University students said "I have always felt that there is a place where

God should dwell, it is not in heaven but in hell". He added after a pause "you see it is there the people require so much of universal love and sympathy". Not many would disagree with this observation if God is accepted to be all merciful and compassionate.

As a devout believer, personally I do not reach Him through the outer trappings and raiments of the church, temples, synagogues, mosques and priesthood. I accept these are a solace to mankind and should be accepted and encouraged as a source of comfort and relief to hundreds of millions, whose lives are otherwise blighted at the stage of being drawers of water and hewers of wood.

It is tragic that God is rarely worshipped in pure esoteric state but only through the medium of superstitions, idolatry, miracles and ecclesiastical dispensations from the pulpit. In India, God is worshipped in a variety of forms and shapes many human, some animals and even trees. Animals such as the monkey, the snake, the elephant, and the cow are objects of veneration. The *peepul (ficus religiosa)* tree is considered sacred and tying strings around its circumference and placing a few stone idols of Hindu gods at the base turns the whole place into a temple and place of worship.

Idolatry abounds amongst 800 million Hindus. One of the important gods in the Hindu pantheon is Lord Ganesha the patron of arts and science and the god of wisdom represented as a figure of elephant and man. He is the son of Shiva and Parvati. He is the eliminator of obstacles and is the god of plenty and bountiful success.

He is worshipped at the beginning of every business venture and at the start of an important journey.

Another deity is Hanuman, the divine monkey, the central figure in the Ramayana (Romance of Rama). He aided Rama in recovering his wife Sita from the demon Ravana. He acted as a spy and when exposed his tail was set on fire and in retaliation he burnt down Lanka. He crossed the straits between Lanka and India in one leap. As a beneficent guardian spirit he is worshipped in the form of a monkey with a red face. He is reckoned to be a model for devotion to god. He is also a popular deity in Japan where there are several Hanuman temples. Lord Shiva, the Creator, representing absolute consciousness, energy, vitality, dynamism and movement in his cosmic dance is all too familiar.

Also Hindus revere snakes and, unless absolutely necessary, it would be a sacrilege to kill one. The cobra, including the King Cobra who can be as long as a New York taxi capable of killing 20 persons with one tea spoon of venom, is held in religious awe.

There is nothing as impressive to the inarticulate millions in India as the supernatural spectacles of gods flying in chariots going to war against evil or in the form of an ape (Hanuman) rescuing a damsel (Sita) in distress abducted by the demon (Ravana). In most cases the allegory demonstrates the triumph of good over evil.

In the name of a deity, cruel rites are also performed including the sacrifice of animals. A revolting rite, which is very rare these days, is the cult of *Sati* which

is the self immolation of the wife on the funeral pyre of her husband to the chanting of hymns, in the midst of hundreds gathered to witness the gruesome spectacle, and then the place where *Sati* is performed is turned into an illegal shrine and temple followed by celebrations and mass gatherings on festival days to propitiate the gods. Sati is a 700 year old custom and was largely practised amongst the warrior community in the beautiful state of Rajasthan. Lord William Bentinck, Governor- General of East India Company, declared it illegal in 1829 and struck it down with an iron fist. The last most talked about *Sati* was in Rajasthan at Deolara village where 18 year old Roop Kanwar immolated herself in 1987 on the funeral pyre of her 25 year old husband Mal Singh. Very recently in August 2009, 60 year old Sharbati Bai attempted to commit sati in Rajasthan's Sikar district but the police stopped her. These rituals, rites and beliefs exist, despite strong opposition from animal and human rights activists, because many of these are the peoples' path to God.

Take another example of belief and faith taken from ancient history. During the Norman conquest of England (1066) a large bright comet was seen in the skies (portrayed in the Bayeux tapestry), which was centuries later identified by Sir Edmond Halley, who charted accurately its course and speed at 80,000 mph (128,000 km). He calculated that it would be visible once in every 76 years and was last seen in November/December 1985. When Julius Caesar died in 44 BC a comet appeared in the sky and the people

of Rome believed that God had sent His chariot to take Caesar's mortal remains to the Heavens!

The waters of the river Ganges (to Indians mother Ganga), which flows from the Himalayas unites with the mighty Brahmaputra(originates in Tibet as the Yarlung Zangbo, the world's highest level river) and empties into the Bay of Bengal creating a 200 miles (320 km.) wide delta, after a journey of 1560 miles (2510 km.), collecting on the way an enormous quantity of industrial effluents, garbage and waste and discarded remains of human corpses. At the holy city of Varanasi (Benares), near Saranath where Gautama Buddha gave his first sermon on enlightenment, thousands of corpses of Hindus are cremated or half cremated (the poor don't have enough money to buy full quantity of wood) and what are left are scattered with ashes on the Ganga. Cremation for the Hindu is necessary for reincarnation of the soul. Water from the Ganga is then sprinkled on the fire from an earthenware pot before it is smashed to mark the release of the soul from the body. In January 2010, millions of people heralded the Maha Kumbh religious fair, which comes every 12 years, by having a dip in the sacred Ganga.

Throughout the year, hundreds of thousands take a holy bath in this heavily polluted river and drink the water and nothing happens to them but it is reckoned drinking is likely to be fatal if one is foolhardy enough to do so a few miles down stream! The Indian Government has now decided to spend $ 3.25 billion for completely cleaning the Ganga so that it is unpolluted and free flowing by

2020 and the exercise will be supported by World Bank assistance of $1 billion

Until a short while ago and even now in parts of Africa the worshippers of inanimate objects were looked upon with pity as "heathens" needing salvation. It may well be asked why should this form of belief be questioned if he is brought nearest to his concept of God. If he is able to reach Him it is good for him. His salvation lies in his belief in God because it mitigates and drowns the harshness of his life and all its disappointments. This contentment is very important for life span.

Also we could question why talk about worshippers of inanimate objects as heathens when the acceptance of "miracles" and "myths" is widespread in the western world amongst Christians who today number more than 1600 million articulated people who are largely free from want. The miracles of Lourdes and Fatima have millions of believers. Sister Lucia dos Santos whose funeral took place in 2005 at age 97, along with Francisco and Jacinta Marto, saw apparitions of Virgin Mary at Fatima in Portugal in 1917 which has become an important Christian shrine in the world visited by thousands of pilgrims annually. In 1930, the children's version of the Lady of the Rosary was officially accepted as the appearance of the Virgin Mary and a basilica was consecrated at the site. Lucia is said to have predicted the end of World War II and the attempted assassination of Pope John Paul II by Mehmet Ali Agca, whom the holy father later pardoned in the prison in the true spirit of Christianity. When these apparitions

were reported 70,000 people gathered at Fatima and saw another "miracle" with the spectacle of the sun moving around veils of silver.

And recently, the apparition of Virgin Mary, marking the death of Pope John Paul II, was claimed to have been seen on the wall of a Chicago subway which was converted into a shrine leading to thousands flocking to the place bearing flowers and candles and clutching rosaries. The apparition was subsequently described as a yellow and white image formed from dripping water mixed with road salts!! The theologians and the believers and the faithful called this a "miracle", the meteorologists called it a weather phenomenon! When millions believe who can question their faith?

The perception of the divinity of Virgin Mary and the crucifixion and resurrection of Jesus Christ are the bedrock of Christianity and you can not be a Christian without believing in Virgin birth and Resurrection although modern thinking is this is not the message of Jesus Christ and is alleged to have been invented much later. This belief, if not myth, is accompanied by mindless bigotry which I personally experienced when a dear friend, who is a recent convert to Christianity, told me seriously that all non-believers, including myself, will rot in hell.

Scientists have tried to question these beliefs, governed as we are by the immutable laws of nature and the conception of birth through the physical union of man and woman and the inevitable finality of mortality. But to the 1600 million Christians they are the most important

tenets of worship with Easter week-- the Resurrection of Jesus Christ—being celebrated by hundreds of millions on the third day of his crucifixion. Easter is central to the whole Christian year as the basis of the Christian faith. Belief in Resurrection is fortified by stories of an empty tomb and apparitions. Nevertheless questions are asked whether these are myths or there is some truth? Is the story of the Exodus to King David and the birth of Jesus Christ also a myth? Does one have to believe in the concept of Virgin Birth and the Resurrection? St. Paul proclaimed "If Christ has not been raised then your faith is futile".

In India devout believers have claimed that the statues of Lord Ganesh and Lord Krishna, two important gods in the Hindu pantheon, actually drank milk leading to mass convergence of worshipers to the temple where this phenomenon had been reported and which was kept open till late into the night. Recently Mumbai witnessed the divine "wedding" of the idols of Lord Balaji and Goddess Padmavati which were brought hundreds of miles from Tirupati in south India. The "wedding" was performed as per Vedic rites in the presence of a mass of devotees. The deluge of miracles and myths has not stopped to beguile the inarticulate believers and Lord Hanuman's idol reportedly shed "tears" in a temple in Mathura several hundred miles south of Mumbai drawing large crowds of devotees.

Are the super natural exploits of the numerous gods of the Hindu pantheon to name a few Ram, Vishnu,

Krishna, Hanuman and others in the conquest of good over evil myths? As an author I have no views to express except to say that all religions have their fair share of myths and miracles and I feel they act as a spark to religion.

In her novel *The Expected One*, Kathleen McGowan claims to be the descendant of Christ on the basis that Mary and Jesus did marry and had children and after 2000 years there would be a large number of their descendants and she claimed to be one of them! It is gathered it was difficult for her to have her book published but later she was sought after as a celebrated author. She is not prepared to reveal whatever evidence she has gathered and it is understood scholars are sceptical of her claims.

To ensure that believers are not weaned away from ecclesiastical beliefs, the General Synod of the Church of England proclaimed some time ago that clergy, who deny the Virgin Birth or the bodily resurrection of Jesus Christ and those who preached liberal doctrine of homosexuality from the pulpit, would be tried as heretics. Apparently, the Church can not now burn the agnostics at the stake as it did in the middle ages which was the fate of Thomas Cranmer, (1489-1556) the first Archbishop of Canterbury and the author of the Book of Common Prayer, who put the English Bible in all the parish churches. He was denounced by Catholic Mary I for propagating Protestantism and was convicted and burnt.

This was a classic case of defiance of religious dogma and there were many others the most prominent being Socrates, the Athenian philosopher, who wrote nothing but

was indicted for corrupting the youth, neglect of the gods, whom the city worshipped, and for practice of religious novelties. He was convicted in BC 399, condemned to death, and given an opportunity to escape but instead drank the fatal hemlock. Also, one of the earliest threats to Vatican rule were the descendents of Cathars, an agnostic sect, to whom true faith meant establishing direct rapport with God without the intervention of the Church and who, on instruction of Pope Innocent III, were ruthlessly massacred in the middle of the 13th century.

It is tragic that most people remember God when they are faced with extreme danger such as the spectre of imminent drowning or an impending air crash or grievous illness. Every human being finds comfort in seeking the hand of Providence. Even atheists and agnostics, if they are lucid at the moment of dire peril, must be invoking the name of God for protection and preservation of life. There is a saying that in combat there are no atheists in a foxhole! It is believed that soldiers in Iraq facing the likelihood of imminent death from unseen hands are believed to have cried out for God--it could be anyone's God as long as the incantation was God-- for redemption and life. Arguably all survivors of earthquakes and similar natural calamities have unreservedly, with few exceptions, admitted owing their lives to a higher being

Ben Sherwood's book "The Survivors Club", relates the amazing survival of one Stan Premnath of new Guyana from the 9/11 holocaust when he witnessed to his horror from the window of his office on the 81st floor

of the South Tower the terrifying sight of a giant aircraft coming straight at him at high speed just before it slammed between the 77th and 85th floor causing vast destruction along with part of the wing wedged into his door 20ft. away but his *Bible was resting on his desk undisturbed*. Prem, who is a church goer but not a religious fanatic, said "the word of God is not destroyed". He cried out "Lord send somebody, anybody. I have two small children! I don't want to die why am I alone? Send someone Lord". He crawled through the devastation and saw the fire warden with a torch and believed this was his guardian angel sent by God in answer to his screams and he survived.

God is also invoked hypocritically. When the British fleet under Lord Nelson, annihilated the French and Spanish fleets at Trafalgar on 6 November, 1805, the despatch announcing the victory read "the attack on them was irresistible, and it pleased the Almighty Disposer of all events to grant His Majesty's arms a complete and glorious victory". Can any thing be more absurd than to imagine that God, in granting victory, was responsible for the deaths of 449 British while, according to British estimates, the enemy lost ten times that number!

We have also examples of royalty and the high and mighty in England congregating in Westminster Abbey in London at the start of World Wars I and II for blessings and for victory in conflicts in which tens of millions were to die with unimaginable devastation and then have thanksgiving prayers when victorious. It is difficult to

accept how highly articulate people invoke God as a tool to protect themselves at the cost of others.

This is not only the negation of faith but also ridicules the greatness of God by seeking His help to cause untold suffering, misery and death. How can He be partisan when the ecclesiastical belief is that He is just and even handed? It would be so much better if the congregation prayed to God to lend a helping hand to bring about peace amongst the warring nations and avoid the inevitable catastrophe brought by devastating wars.

Can one be a good scientist and believe in God? This question was raised at a scientific conference at a City College in New York. It was said that belief in the supernatural, especially belief in God, was incompatible with good science. However, disdain for belief in god was far from universal amongst the scientists gathered and those amongst them, who were religious minded, spoke out saying that religion and science were two separate domains.

In 2009 on the bicentenary of Charles Darwin, who is acclaimed to be in the same league as a scientist with Newton and Einstein, there was extensive discussion on the great divide between science and religion. In 1859 Darwin, on the publication of his epoch making *On the Origin of Species by Means of Natural Selection*, shook ecclesiastical belief by his well considered documented theory of evolution and the descent of Man which was contrary to the church belief that the universe was too complicated to invent itself and was the work

of the Creator. This doctrine of Intelligent Design, as an alternative to Darwin's natural selection, has a wide following in USA where, in some schools, the teachings of Darwin are proscribed in favour of the fundamentalist ID doctrine.

Powerful voices in the Vatican called for calm and have asserted that science and religion have different fields in which to perform their roles. When greeting noted astrophysicist Stephen Hawking at a meeting of scientific academicians at the Vatican, Pope Benedict XVI said "There is no opposition between faith's understanding of creation and the evidence of the empirical sciences" and added "Galileo saw nature as a book whose author is God"! A short while ago, the Dalai Lama, at a conference on Science and Spirituality in New Delhi, emphasised that religion and spirituality should accept something conclusively proved by science even if it goes against traditional views.

Recently one Luigi Cascioli, who studied for priesthood, but becoming very disillusioned turned into a militant atheist has, in his book *The Fall of Christ*, questioned that all claims for Jesus Christ's historical existence, other than the Bible, rely on authors who lived after the "hypothetical" Christ and thus were not reliable witnesses to the belief that He lived and died in Palestine in the 1st century.

For the impoverished, belief and faith are strong *mantras* and it is difficult to argue when they take a strong hold on the mind. People's faith is aesthetic, ethical and

inspirational with religion acting as a source of moral foundation. Faith, religion and prayers are the three most powerful survival invocations. They will bury all your demons and bring stability and peace during difficult times. Even if they do not help you to survive physically in times of great stress they would bring to you a kind of inner peace and mental fortitude which will act to relieve any tragedy facing you. Martin Luther said "Faith must trample under foot all reason, sense and understanding". Faith is not even the last to die.

My personal belief in God is supported with the regular power of prayers shorn of all kinds of supernatural myths which gives me great calm and peace to face all the vicissitudes and stress of life. I start and end the day with prayers which are totally devoid of asking for any favours for myself and my family. To the reader I commend strongly this way of life.

A recent preliminary research study, undertaken by the University of Chicago, to determine the relationship between religious disposition and health, indicated that belief in God improves a person's physical well-being. A Texas University study on power of religion on longevity concluded that regular church goers live about seven years longer than those who do not. Recently, the Archbishop of Westminster, in his pastoral letter to his diocese, mentioned that stable, fruitful and healthy lives cannot be achieved without daily prayer which is essential for our well-being. It is unarguable that life span depends in a large measure on spiritual contentment brought about

by belief in God and the power of prayers and, other things being equal, by physical condition, mental alacrity, moderation in consumption of food and drinks and a disciplined life style free from excesses.

There is appalling poverty and distress in some of the Asian and African countries and India. In life a charitable disposition sharing one's wealth, time and expertise with the needy, the poor, the disadvantaged, would lead to great spiritual enlightenment and mental satisfaction promoting a long life span. I know of missionaries in the service of Christ, leaving the comfort of their homes and life style, settling far away from their developed societies and spending their future life, along with their families, in some of the most inhospitable places in the world, particularly in Africa and India. They are devoted to doing admirable work in education, social uplift, medical care, agriculture, animal husbandry and similar causes for the poor and the needy. Some of them follow in the footsteps of their fathers and forefathers, going to economically undeveloped areas in harsh climate, leading a Spartan life of denial and self abnegation, living simply and eating basic food not far from what is eaten by the poor whom they are selflessly serving. They are exposed to painful and debilitating illnesses.

This is real devotion to God sacrificing all that is comfortable and enjoyable in their lives to ameliorate the condition of the unwanted and the disadvantaged. Albert Einstein truly said "Only a life lived for others is the life worthwhile." As an example there is much to

commend the renowned work done in parts of rebellious, unruly, inhospitable Africa by Médicines sans Frontière, a French mission, largely consisting of dedicated young specialists.

Jimmy Carter, the former President of United States, known for his humanitarian work for the poor and downtrodden, organised building of safe, simple, liveable homes for the poor near Lonavala, a holiday resort at an elevation of 1800 ft. situated 80 miles from Mumbai, under Habitat for India a Jimmy Carter Work Project. This endeavour attracted many high profile individuals, including it is understood Brad Pitt, from all over the world to contribute to the social cause. This was followed by the Jimmy Carter Habitat project in Thailand in December 2009 with 3000 volunteers drawn from all over the world to build 82 homes in 7 days in celebration of the 82nd birthday of the King.

It is reported that a 26 year old Australian is all set to run a full marathon every day for 40 days to complete the journey from Mumbai to Bangalore in India, a distance of 1300 kms, to raise money for a school for poor children of quarry workers and thus alleviate their grinding poverty. He will be running through mountains, forests and coffee plantations. What will lead him to embark on this venture has been the horrendous conditions of the quarry workers who work for 12 hours a day 6 days in a week breaking hard rock with a hammer.

There can be no greater satisfaction in our lives than to share our wealth with those in need of help. In the last

century, the industrial revolution created enormous wealth for some. The rich became incredibly richer, the poor dismally poorer. Vast fortunes were made. Rockefeller, who amassed his wealth in oil, established an original foundation of $100 million nearly a century ago in 1919, a sum which would be equivalent to several billions in today's money. Carnegie, who substituted undependable iron with cheap steel, was even more generous donating $300 million at about the same time. He said "the man who dies rich dies disgraced".

Rockefeller was supposed to have been told by his almoner Frederick Gates that if he did not give his money to charity "it will crush you and your children and your grandchildren". It was Rockefeller who said "God gave me my money. I believe the power to make money is a gift from God to be developed and used to the best of our ability for the good of mankind. Having been endowed with the gift I possess, I believe it is my duty to make money and still more money and to use the money I make for the good of my fellow man according to the dictates of my conscience."

In our century, Bill Gates, estimated to be the richest man on the planet, established in 2000 the Bill and Melinda Gates Foundation (net worth $29 billion), which is the international leader particularly in the war against HIV, tuberculosis and malaria in poorest parts of Africa and India. It provides 90% of world's budget for eradication of polio and has committed $1.5 billion to Global Alliance for Vaccines and Immunisation (GAVI)

for helping children in poor countries who cannot afford vaccines. TIME magazine praised the Foundation for "giving more money away faster than anyone ever has".

Recently Gates visited some of the poorest parts of India which he humorously dubbed "with the least amount of drinking water and most amount of sun" and was very agreeably surprised that immunisation rates had shot up from 11% to 60%. He eulogised the life saving effects of vaccination by remarking that 20 million children died in 1960 but in 2009 the deaths were reduced to 9 million due to the miracle of vaccination. His foundation has given India $ 1 billion alone for health projects.

The world's second richest individual Warren Buffet, the Chairman of Berkshire Hathway, is reported to have given 99% of his massive wealth reckoned to be about $ 46 billion to charity. Gates and Buffet have now embarked on an enterprise to persuade their super rich friends to donate at least half of their fortunes to charity. The campaign called The Giving Pledge with a minimum target of $600 billion has received encouraging response. Buffet and Gates are very close friends and the former has said publicly that Gates is the smartest guy he has ever met.

Narayan Murthy, the father of India's software development, has truly said that the real power of money is the power to give it away. *INFOSYS* founded by Murthy, is the second largest IT organisation in India quoted on *NASDAQ*. He is deeply involved in the field of hospitals, orphanages, scientific centres, schools and libraries and

is a strong advocate of what he calls "compassionate capitalism".

We are all reward driven creatures belonging to the maniacal age of materialism whose god is acquisition, greed, and acquiring power by fair or foul means. Greed brings in its train tainted success or acute disappointment from failure shortening life through stress, tension, fear, cardiac disorders and a host of other physical problems. Contentment so essential for a long life span becomes a stranger and there is no fulfilment in life if you are not able to share what you have with the poor and the disadvantaged even if it means you have to go without something you want. Even a small contribution from your income to deserving causes for people less fortunate than yourself will bring love of a different kind into your life and uplift your human psyche giving immense satisfaction. After all you may not need all the money you earn and sharing a part of it is not going to make a dent in your life style.

Chapter II

**"Retirement is the ugliest word
in the English language"
Earnest Hemingway**

Profound Influence of Mind on Life Span

Mind and its alacrity have the most profound influence in shaping the life of human beings. If the mind dims it dims the light in life. The process of degeneration then becomes irreversible and no amount of medical assistance will restore it to its original state. It is the absolute captain in total command of the ship of life. It is the prime motivator of all human actions and achievements. How often have we heard "it is all in the mind" when describing any achievement or lack of it in the sports field particularly when playing games. Thought processes play a very important role in how one plays and the excellence achieved. Mechanics and technique are useful up to a point but the engine which drives technique is the brain.

Survival in times of acute distress and disappointments in life are all in the mind.

Mind is as important and precious as the life saving function of the heart. It controls and has destiny over your health and body. It is claimed by recent scientific research that even pain can be wished away by manipulating the brain. More and more people are becoming increasingly aware of the domination of the mind over the body as a support for a long healthy life.

There is a tendency amongst those who have reached retirement at 60/65 to pay least attention to capsule the mind to keep it vibrant and active. From friends who have retired, it is quite usual to hear "I enjoy my life in total relaxation without a care in the world". This is the surest prescription for rapid decline and incapacity and earlier than normal mortality. Reaching 60/65 and above is a critical time in one's existence and should be grasped and challenged as a new chapter in life full of constructive activity, resurgence and happiness.

Take the case of one Mr. Hall who suffered cerebral oedema in May 2006 after successfully scaling Mount Everest. His companions, after struggling valiantly for hours whilst descending to bring him to safety, reluctantly abandoned him for dead stripping him of all his equipment including oxygen. After some hours he woke up in total darkness nearly buried in snow in biting cold and without much of his life saving equipment suffering from hypothermia, hypoxia (lack of oxygen) etc. Determined to stay alive he tenaciously went through the

night resolutely focusing his mind on survival and tackled what was impossible. When he was ultimately rescued he was barely clothed and had spent the night at 8600m. without oxygen coming out alive after an incredible feat. Later Hall said staying alive was a great motivator and I just tackled what was impossible "keeping the mind ticking over, putting it all together".

Other instances are the 13 year old girl who was rescued after 12 hours from a plane crash, which killed all 152, by clinging to a piece of wreckage and the three Chinese coal miners rescued after 25 days trapped underground during which they licked moisture trickling down the walls. Ben Sherwood in his book "The Survivor's Club" writes "My thesis is that survival is a mindset, it's a lens, it's an outlook".

From a life full of activity you are suddenly confronted on retirement with the fact of having nothing to do. The changed attitude is that a new life is opening up for luxuriating with a little bit of pottering in the garden, angling, occasional round of golf, watching TV, exchanging banter and gossip at the local or at coffee meetings with friends. Generally speaking, the tendency will be to baulk at any activity which will keep the mind on a sharp edge. By taking life easily both physically and mentally is the surest way to fade into oblivion.

On retirement a mind set must be developed that advancing years are not going to cramp your life style. A determined action path must be laid to ensure that age does not dog and dominate your life even at a subconscious

level. Swat the fear of ageing as you would swat a fly and develop a mental attitude that will defeat the belief that you are old. The mind must be made to work to din into you that advancing age is not a disease but a new type of deliverance. Be resolute enough to face the reality of old age which is the period where you must never feel there is nothing to focus on except illness and death. The last two have lived with us as a reality since our birth and should not cause any fear.

Early results of research conducted in US indicate that mental stimulation can go a long way as protection against Alzheimer disease and dementia. In the US, brain health programmes including "brain gymnasiums" and "brain healthy" foods are spreading offering fountain of youth. MetLife is pushing brain health by providing brain fitness software to millions of older customers. Web sites like Happyneuron.com and MyBrainTrainer.com describing cranial callisthenics have been developed offering possibilities of quicker and sharper mental responses

Like every part of the body it is most important for older people to exercise the brain to improve cognitive abilities, memory, reasoning and speed thinking. Treat the brain as a muscle and exercise it as you would exercise the muscles of your body to keep the body vibrant and strong. This will increase ability to perform daily functions including financial matters without reliance on others. Learn to play bridge and Su Doku and indulge in these past times. Do simple calculations by mental arithmetic. Responses then will be sharp and quick and

the biological process of degeneration of the brain will be arrested delaying memory loss and dementia which are the curse of old age.

On retirement lying on a hammock or garden chair or watching a ball game and soaps on TV until your eyelids struggle to remain open are the surest early passage to physical and mental disability. For reading by all means keep next to you Tom Clancy, Dan Brown, D.H. Lawrence but also throw in classical mythology like Homer's epic (*The Iliad and the Odyssey*), elementary mathematics, Shakespeare, natural histories, biographies, great travels and explorations. Apart from giving immense pleasure, this type of quality reading will sharpen and widen the mind and keep it in a state of constant alertness.

To keep the mind on razor's edge read what is difficult to assimilate even if it means reading a part once over for better comprehension. I have always made it a point to read difficult and absorbing texts, although at times this has driven me to tears, but the knowledge that is acquired and its recantation at the end of the day is a sublime pleasure. When I recommend reading difficult subjects, I am not advocating the reading of Sanskrit grammar or Albert Einstein's *Theory of Relativity* or Newton's *Principia* or Robert Cannibal's *The Man Who Knew Infinity* (life of mathematical genius Ramanujan) though the last book even for a layman is fascinating and interesting reading.

Then it is very important to guard against depression, basically a mood disorder, which transforms personality, resulting in losing interest in what is going on in life,

a feeling of hopelessness, irritability, despondence, reluctance to communicate even with family members, loss of appetite and libido. It can strike anyone at any stage. Women are prone to it due to hormonal changes on menopause and childbirth. Also, not living in the thick of activity can be acutely depressing.

Mostly everyone suffers from some state of depression brought about by loss of a job, business not doing well facing losses, mounting debts with lack of ability to pay off, marital problems with the marriage on which so much reliance was put going down hill or disappointment in a fresh love interest. Depression being self- limiting with proper counselling, medically supervised use of anti-depressants and family support is likely to disappear and if it is a passing phenomenon, as in most cases, it holds no terrors. However, a permanent mood disorder could lead to grave consequences. It can be devastating to personal health, affecting family life, lowering energy levels, work performance and even result in impotence. In extreme instances, it can lead to suicidal and homicidal tendencies as demonstrated by the suicide of Germany's celebrated football international who threw himself in front of a train. No amount of counselling by professionals and steadfast compassion and understanding of his wife could prevent his suicidal mission.

Increasingly depressed people are advised to take to "mindfulness" treatment which essentially is meditation with "thought training" reducing reliance on anti-depressants. Mindfulness is based on eastern philosophy

particularly Budhism where the mind is taught to focus on one issue rejecting all the daily worrying chores plaguing the mind.

Leading a life of a widower for nearly 50 years with my daughters and grandchildren away, I have had my moments of depression caused by loneliness and also due to my inability to participate in physical activities as I used to due to lack of youthful energy. When I watch cricket, football, golf, in none of which I excelled, I am nostalgically reminded of playing these games with great gusto and pleasure. I played competitive golf until I was 75, with a handicap which became gradually depressing with advancing age, but now my legs groan walking a full round (moving in golf carts knocks the pleasure out of golf which is walking on verdant grass and negotiating the gradients of the course).

I envy the young whenever I see them running up and down the stairs which I used to do once and which is now beyond me. I face the reality of physical limitation and do not fight against it. When the World's oldest man Henry Allingham, the only survivor of the First World War who died recently after celebrating his 113th birthday, was asked about his exceptional longevity, replied "I don't know if there is a secret but keeping within your capacity is vital…..the trick is to look after yourself and always know your limitations".

I am also frustrated that I am not participating in any capacity in the fast growing economic development of India. I see fundamental changes in industrial and

corporate management and practices and I am overcome with remorse that I am playing no part in it. I miss the excitement, the frenetic activity, the risk taking in management decisions, the seminars, the conviviality of meeting other businessmen and planning for the better future of India and its people. As I have broadened my mental and occupational horizons I have not allowed this alienation to put me down.

Anyone living in India, with a modicum of sensitivity and compassion for the poor and the horribly undernourished, cannot help being overcome with acute frustration in the environment in which one lives. After 63 years of Independence, which brought with it self-rule, India still ranks 127 out of 177 countries on the UN Development Index which includes, education, health care, living standards and life span. Children and adolescents are as thin as sticks. Visit any playground in India and you will see unarguably the thinnest school going children and college students on the planet. A UNICEF report records India has the highest number of malnourished kids in the world --about 57 million-- or more than one-third of the world's 147 million.

In the population of 1100 millions, there are tens of millions who are called adivasis, tribals and "dalits" (previously known as the untouchables to the Brahmins) until social reformers fought and gave them the right to exist with pride and dignity. But they still remain very backward and all the government talk of inclusive economic and social development has barely reached them

even on the fringes leading to violent activists creating mayhem under Mao's banner.

With their empowerment as a large voting power, present day governments have awakened to the need to improve their lot by building schools, hospitals and imparting basic skills in centres established in even remote areas so that they can take their rightful place in Indian society. But the effort is so minimal that in some areas 150 children study and sleep in same room. In other parts the budget for their food is US 50 cents per day per student and consequently the gap between meals is heartrending and is broken by a snack or two. In one school they have a breakfast of eggs, sprouts, bananas but no wash room and have to go to the nearest river to bathe. Development is seeping through and the country can now boast of having had a Dalit as one of the past Presidents of India and also another, until recently, was the Chief Justice of the Supreme Court.

Because of inadequate diet, children's physical stature is not up to any worthwhile standards for excellence in sports, except in cricket. In the past several years I do not remember India making any mark at World Olympics, except winning a gold in hockey several years ago, in shooting recently and otherwise very few bronze and silver. We are so starved of sporting achievements that any individual winning gold in the World Olympics

(a rarest of rare event) is instantly made a hero and an icon. A girl, who used to be about 50 in singles tennis ranking and is near 100 now, was dubbed "tennis

sensation" with a reputed income of a few million dollars in endorsements. Only one golfer has broken the top 50 barrier. Our world ranking in rugby was somewhere around 83 because there are so many Ophelias in the team who look Lilliputians as compared to international players. In football, India was about 177 in FIFA ranking.

It is claimed that there is no starvation in India which is true, as compared to the great Bengal Famine in the early 1940s during the Second World War, when quantities of staples like rice and wheat were sent by the British rulers to the North African and Middle Eastern theatres of war along with a large number of railway rolling stock creating acute shortage and disrupting movement of relief supplies.

But starvation deaths are still reported every year on a small scale from isolated pockets of rural communities due to crippling indebtedness arising from failure of crops following inadequate rainfall and uneconomical support prices for crops. Government pulls out all stops to give assistance by wiping off debts, extending liberal credit, injecting purchasing power into the hands of the impoverished peasantry and giving them basic employment.

This is done under a government administered Employment Guarantee Relief scheme giving farmers staples with a cash handout of about a little more than one US dollar a day which, by the time the poor unemployed worker receives for a day's hard work, is reduced to about US 80 cents by corrupt intermediaries and bureaucrats

who make a killing. The scheme has been wrecked by widespread corruption. Government audit has revealed that out of the annual budget of $8.33 billion, a whopping 40% has been siphoned off by administrators in the rural areas.

Mr. Paul Wolfowitz, the former neo- conservative deputy secretary of defence in the Bush administration, and subsequently during his brief term as the President of the World Bank, waged a relentless war against corruption suspending millions of dollars of aid sanctioned for some countries whose record left much to be desired. He is on record saying the Bank's mission "was to send children to school, to help mothers be healthier, to provide jobs for poor people and not have resources siphoned of into the hands of the corrupt and greedy". He suspended $ 800 millions in loans for maternal and children's health care in India on discovering that relief payments were gobbled up by officials.

India is home to the world's largest concentration of the poor. Poverty in India and accompanying wretchedness has no impact in cold print. You have to be in the midst of it and see it and yours eyes will well up with tears. An important plank of government is to reduce and eventually eradicate poverty, but these are rhetorical statements and action has been abysmally slow despite Five year economic development plans in the past 63 years of self- rule.

The late Mrs. Indira Gandhi fought and won a national election by a landslide, by cleverly coining the rabble rousing slogan *Garibi Hatao* (remove poverty),

which caught the imagination of the poor inarticulate electorate. Now the New Age politicians have gone better and are offering cleverly *roti, bijlee, pani, makan, sadak* (food, electricity, water, homes and roads) to capture the minds of the gullible electorate. Political parties in the 2009 General Elections went one better by offering a wide range of freebees such as free electricity, TV set, rent free housing, highly subsidised food grains, clothing and the like despite existing governments being already totally impoverished and bankrupt.

Indeed the task of economic development is of Himalayan proportions defeated by bureaucratic inertia, wastages, monumental corruption and the inexorable increase in population (about 22 million are added every year equal to the population of Australia), which diminishes the per capita income, despite the current annual economic growth rate of about 7% (second only to China) and a domestic savings rate of up to 30%.

In Mumbai city out of an estimated population of 14 millions only 50% live in apartments and constructed structures. The remaining urban poor live, raise families and die on pavements, in improvised hutments or in dilapidated structures in abominable conditions lacking adequate water supply and sanitation. In the midst of this grinding poverty and horrible living conditions is it believable that a new high rise coming up in down town Mumbai is believed to cost $2 billion. But this is India where the gulf between the very rich and the poor is as wide as the Pacific Ocean and nobody cares.

The rich continue to indulge in a vulgar display of wealth by staging the most outrageously lavish wedding receptions hosting feasts for thousands of well fed rich guests in mind boggling spectacles. Whole mock replicas of India's famous palaces and temples are set up for one day's festivities at enormous cost. The very rich families indulge in one up-man-ship to outdo others at a time when the poor are hopefully waiting outside to collect scraps. It brings to mind the pot bellied characters in Charles Dickens's *Oliver Twist* who gorge themselves on choice cuts of beef Wellington while Oliver helplessly asks for more gruel.

Marriages in India are a serious drain on the pockets of the poor. In every marriage traditionally gold ornaments play an important part and have to be exchanged. The poorest peasant will borrow money at even usurious interest rate to purchase ornaments. This is why India continues to be one of the world's largest consumers of gold reckoned at about 400/500t per annum.

The rich and the super rich continue to spend their lives in a rarefied monetary atmosphere. Buying automobiles costing up to a quarter million dollars and gifting a multi million dollar pleasure yacht as birthday gift are all ugly demonstration of wealth in a country, where 400 millions live below the line of poverty earning a dollar a day. The situation will worsen as according to a joint report by the Wold Bank and IMF, 782 million will be living on less than $2 a day by 2015. Poverty in India has no dimensions. It is reported that thousands of women in India in agricultural

communities, due to chronic malnutrition and extreme poverty, reach menopause between 30/34 which is truly a very sad state of affairs.

This abject disregard for the poor relapses an individual into a state of acute despair praying upon the mind. After all what can he do except feel utterly helpless. The saddest part is that there is little or no awareness amongst the rich to lend a helping hand on a large institutional scale to eradicate poverty. Indian cities are bursting with millionaires with many reputed to be worth billions in dollar terms. Additionally it is reckoned that hundreds of millions are stashed away in foreign tax heavens. No one has thought yet of starting The Giving Pledge enterprise of Bill Gates and Warren Buffet. There is no call to arms by energising the people of India and its corporations to launch a crusade with the pro-active participation of Government. It seems everyone has become inured to poverty's presence.

There are some selfless individuals who have done remarkable charitable and social work in India amongst the poor which is limited in its reach. A very significant social activist who has dedicated her life to speak and fight for the poor is Medha Patkar of India. A young girl she has now aged before her time with greying hair due to occasional fasting and deprivation to protect the poorest who are evacuated by force by land sharks or government agencies from their shanties with the latter sometimes providing them with alternate accommodation. Recently 3500 shanties were bulldozed on the fringes of Mumbai

city throwing out the poor inhabitants without a roof but Medha was there, if unable to stop the carnage, at least counselling, giving solace and wiping off their tears. She waged a relentless non-violent battle to delay the dispossession of land of hundreds of farmers when the mighty Narmada dam was constructed to secure for them adequate compensation and suitable alternate land.

Can poverty be made history? Nobel Laureate Mohammed Yunus of Bangladesh, in his acceptance speech for the Nobel Peace Prize at Stockholm on 10 December 2006, said this mission is possible "We will create a poverty museum in 2030". Yunus celebrated as a banker to the poor by lending US $800 million to 7 million impoverished Bangladeshis without collateral with 99 % repayment record has become a legend in his country and famous in the world.

Addressing a summit of 150 world leaders at the UN on 14 September 2005, Mr. George W. Bush, the former President of USA, is reported to have given a clarion call to "tear down the walls" between the rich and poor nations and added "there can be no safety in looking away or seeking the quiet life by ignoring the hardship and oppression of others".

I have elaborated at length on poverty, corruption, ostentatious display of wealth, inadequate nourishment of the youth of India because it is agonising to enjoy a life style which is way above what the poor eke out. When I sit down at the table to eat or go to sleep in a climate controlled room on a comfortable bed I am constantly

reminded of the tens of millions, including infants and children, going to sleep on a hungry stomach and on hard dirty pavements infested with vermin and rats. As an individual I am helpless since, what is required is not charity in bits and pieces, but vast governmental and institutional effort.

Unless one lacks sensitivity and is heartless what is seen and experienced in India deeply affects physical and mental outlook. I am living my long life in this despairing environment and I just cannot wish it away as none of my business or brood like Achilles in my tent. My strong vibrant mind battles forces of depression and angst, which attack from all sides, otherwise I would be mentally disoriented. The fact that I have survived in this environment to reach 92 is a testimony to the disciplines I have elaborated for a long healthy life which are worth practicing.

Chapter III

**"Human beings are like wine
some turn to vinegar
the best improve with age"**

Ageing and the Way to its Conquest

In Jacobean times 45 was a geriatric age. Now with the advent and advance of medical care and the increasing awareness for physical fitness, even generals, past their 60s, have led vast armies into battle. Large industrial and corporate conglomerates are headed by men and women well into their 60s. There is nothing like mid-life crisis. When age 60 is reached, the mind must be set to focus on what should be done in the next 10, 20, 30 years.

Treat 60 as the way to the new 80. Do not entertain negative thoughts that age and death are soon going to consume you. At this landmark the curtain does not fall. There is nothing like enjoying the power you wield at this age with your position and status, vast experience,

connectivity, and adequate resources freeing you from want, if your finances have been well managed.

In economically developed countries getting old now is not as daunting as it was in the earlier part of the last century. The aged are enjoying the best of times with larger families and grandchildren, ease of mobility, revolution in communications, home entertainment, and comfortable homes for the old with pensions and other social security benefits. Nevertheless, though respected, they are somewhat marginalised, sometimes looked upon patronisingly and shunted from the mainstream of society leading to loss of confidence at home, in the community and at the work place.

Are you daunted by age? Well let me write about a person who has had a heart bye-pass some years ago, is known to be afraid of heights, has had prostate cancer treatment, has lost several toes to frostbite, is an internationally acclaimed explorer (Guiness World Records calls him the world's greatest living adventurer), has led the first polar circumnavigation of the earth, has reached both the North and South Poles and, after the bye-pass, has run 7 consecutive marathons in 7 days in 7 countries defying jet lags and, of all desires burning within him, ventured in 2005 after the bye-pass to climb Mount Everest by the dangerous North Face route where the intense cold could cause deadly pulmonary oedema. In his quest, he came very near to reaching the peak but at about 28,100 ft., just short by 800ft., he had to give up because his heart gave a warning alert.

Refusing to be daunted he conquered Everest subsequently. Is it believable that Sir Ranulph Fiennes, with indomitable courage, which at age 67 had not diminished, was fired by adventure to reach the peak where the oxygen content in the air is only 6% and raised £ 3 million ($ 4.80 million) for charity? His second marriage honeymoon was at Base Camp but is alleged to have turned out to be a drip for lack of privacy.

Lord Attenborough, one of the world's greatest naturalist and conservationist, has reached the South Pole and now at age 83 is planning an attempt on the North Pole

Henry Kissinger is a shining study of a man with a sparkling mind, erudition and wide international strategic vision, who is a well known author, chronicler of Castlereagh and Metternich, who opened the China window for Richard Nixon, the former President of United States, and a speaker who can hold his audience spell bound on a geopolitical subject (I heard him speak in Mumbai). Bernard Kouchner, the former UN Commissioner for Kosovo and now Foreign Minister of France, is reported to have said that for Europe he is truly one of the last wise man. No door is closed to him in the higher echelons of Governments and he is now about 85.

Sir John Mills, the famous British actor, who died at age 97, was active in his 90s and played the part of a comedian in Stephen Fry's "Bright Young Things in 2003." A 67 year old British bull fighter, with rickety

knees and aged heart, entered the bull ring near Malaga in Spain in end August last year.

Simon Murray, 63, from Bath became the oldest person to walk 690 miles across the icy wastelands in temperature as low as - 35C to reach the South Pole in January 2004.

I refer to the path making feat of Padampat Singhania, a leading Indian industrialist who, at age 67, broke the world record of high altitude hot air balloon on 26 November 2005 by reaching 69,852 ft., almost on the fringes of space (70,000 ft.), over the coast of western India and beat the 17 year old record held by Per Linstrand by 5,000 ft. He did not wear any space suit but piloted the balloon in a specially made pressurised capsule. Both the camera and radio communication systems failed and all his excitement and joy on reaching the near extremity of space have been lost to posterity. He attempted to touch "the face of God" at a height where the outside temperature was -93 C with negligible oxygen levels.

Unlike most couples, Ken and Marcia Powers of USA, 60 and 58 years of age, did not quietly drift into retirement and early mortality. They meticulously and logistically planned and executed in 2005 a hike of 4900 miles in 235 days starting from Lake Henlopen, Delaware and ending at Point Reyes, California. They walked through 8 States, out wearing 10 pairs of shoes, experiencing freezing snow, quicksand, sandstorms before reaching their destination and naturally losing weight. At the end, they declared they felt fine and somewhat sad that their great odyssey

was over. Their 30 year marriage was the ultimate winner. There was no mid-life crisis and at age 60 a new life of adventure had bugged them.

These instances are related to emphasise what people can do in their mid- life and "so called old age" if they are physically fit, mentally alert and have a positive attitude. If you have an innovative mind you will suddenly find new things to engage your attention and fruitfully occupy your time. You may want to paint or draw sketches bringing out latent artistic talent or engage in social work by teaching others your professional skills thus enhancing the fabric of life style of the community you are living in, learn new skills or languages, write a biography or write on any other subject which interests you spending time on research, go on a geographical expedition. The possibilities are wide ranging if only you will focus your mind.

According to researchers from the Institute of Psychiatry at the Maudsley Hospital, London active occupation delays the onset of dementia which could well be at the rate of one month for every year of work. Actually, it is believed the UK government is thinking of advancing the retirement age from 65 to 70 but this is to assist management of the national debt which will indirectly postpone Alzheimer disease if the above research is effective.

Do not be alarmed if the muscles begin to groan and crick. As you grow older the muscles in your body slowly lose their ability to regenerate resulting in loss of strength and agility. A study of muscle samples of healthy men and

women at a famous US clinic identified that the DNA in our muscles start deteriorating from age 30, and that is why our limbs begin to groan as we grow older. This may be arrested by aerobic exercises and gymnasium work.

Next to a sharp mind, physical fitness, which is currently and correctly the buzzword, is very important for a long life span. A daily brisk walk of at least 4 to 5 km. in not more than 45 minutes is an absolute must. The time taken can be gradually increased with advancing age. To the extent possible, the walk should be completed without a chattering companion remembering that a glass of whisky tastes better when enjoyed in silence. Walking, does not tax the heart, has the salutary effect of burning calories, increasing blood level functions, metabolising food, reducing the incidence of colds and prevents the risk of osteoporosis, which is the curse of old age. Walking as an exercise to reduce weight is misleading, even if it is a daily power walk, though it may maintain weight at an unchanged level and is good as a lung opener and for stamina.

Swimming is not a weight losing exercise. Contrary to accepted belief a work out in gymnasium is not weight reducing though it will tone the body, add muscle and make you feel fitter. I have yet to come across anyone claiming that gymnasium work has led to perceptible weight reduction unless accompanied by conscientious dieting. Fanned by high pressure publicity, a work out in gymnasiums has become a part of life particularly of the elite but this is welcome for fitness.

I repeat again most importantly never lose an opportunity to walk, if not too far, to fetch newspapers and groceries, to post a letter, to visit your banker, to purchase odds and ends and to visit the local. It will not reduce your weight but it will do a world of good by burning calories and tone and keep your body in shape. Frankly, I am now hard put to complete a daily 4 km. walk which I was used to but resolutely I try half the distance and make my legs carry me without fail even in the heat of summer, with its energy sapping humidity which reaches up to 85 %, and when it pours during the monsoon from June to September. The mild muscular pain, the ache in the legs, the sweating followed by a cold shower are exhilarating.

Jogging, if medically allowed, may be helpful in reducing weight. For those in their 60s, jogging, field games like rugby, football, cricket, basketball, riding, lifting heavy weights should be all taboo. A not too vigorous set or two of tennis need not be harmful. There is no need to foolishly over stretch fading physical prowess. Control your impulses and self belief that you can do more. Pay great respect to limitations imposed by age. If you get out of sync with reality you will wind up being dissociated with the future. Remember you want to embark on an odyssey which will make your life worth living instead of developing bed sores or reaching early mortality.

Also in old age do not be under any delusion that you possess the energy and enthusiasm of a teenager or can enjoy a string of mistresses like Picasso, who at 70, was

known to stub cigarettes on their cheeks without murmur or dissent and being rich and famous got away with it. A woman past her 60 should not aspire to be Violetta (*Verdi's La Traviata*) singing and seducing men with the face masked by a fan. Let me quote Horace "Not yours the dance band and the red rose nor the cask drained to its last drag, you are an old woman now." Nor should an aged man think he is Leander swimming the Hellespont daily to meet his lover Hero until he drowns on a stormy night.

Age is no friend to the over reaching. Respect your age and do not bounce like a puppy. Act your age in presence, behaviour and conversation and observe how attractive you make yourself. With age comes so much power to influence people, financial independence to satisfy your personal needs and to be looked at respectfully. You are really in the comfort zone enjoying life if you are fit and healthy.

In India and that goes for most south east Asian countries, most affluent families have extra help to perform a number of functions such as cleaning the apartment, cooking, waiting on the table, chauffeurs to drive cars and valets running errands, including fetching a glass of water or preparing and serving tea, all involving physical exertions. This help is affordable and readily available though times are perceptibly changing. In India a live-in cook, valet and maid (available any time of the day and night) and chauffeur would cost no more than $ 800/1000 per month. What price, what luxury!

This is not sweated labour but much needed employment of skills in a country where, by the latest count of the International Labour Office, there are nearly 40 million unemployed. (In a recent notice by India's largest public sector bank a million applicants applied for 11000 vacancies!) In a tropical country this assistance may be considered necessary and helpful but employment of domestic help means the employer is not utilising his energy which could be harnessed and put to good use to keep fit. It is like water escaping from an inadequately closed tap.

Why waste money on gymnasium, exercise bikes, tread mills and other related equipment when your own home, as one writer put it, is an "Aladdin's cave of DIY exercise equipment". For women who are not professionally career bound, the floor cleaning mop, the vacuum cleaner, the clothes washer, pillow punching and ironing board are all friends for burning excess calories and attaining high level of fitness. Some women do not take kindly to this type of domestic work and treat it as demeaning remaining physically unfit. This is the great advantage of living in the west as domestic help is expensive and you are forced to spend physical energy. Scientists have discovered that life span can be extended if one does not shirk household chores.

Leonie Bloomfield, an expert in time management, following a study carried out at Victoria University, Melbourne, has said having too much time to kill can be deadly for men. "It is clear that having more free

time—and men already enjoy more than women because of gender inequalities in housework, child care and other unpaid work—does not guarantee a leisure experience or better health. Men suffer more chronic conditions; have higher death rates at all ages and account for most causes of death and die, on average, six years younger. It might be worth while to exchange some of their leisure for higher participation in domestic work".

As long as there is mental alertness and reactions are sharp with good eyesight do continue with driving which is a very pleasurable mental exercise. I have not baulked at driving in Mumbai with a million cars, many of them in unserviceable condition, all jockeying without discipline for space on roads built for not more than 50,000 cars. The traffic is horrendous and is zany, tortuous with cars, ancient taxis and several hundred thousand motor cycles all zooming past, cutting and overtaking hazardously, as if there is no tomorrow and they are on the Indianapolis circuit.

There are tens of thousands of two wheelers with infants and children precariously perched on the laps of parents who, along with the police, have least regard for the safety and lives of the young ones who given one nudge in the undisciplined traffic would send the whole family to the undertaker's door. Life is indeed cheap what with nearly 1100 million people to spare! Then there is the gauntlet to be faced with thousands of jay walkers darting across the road with not a care in the world and with no sense of survival. Of course, there are zebra crossings for

pedestrians but neither the drivers nor the police care two hoots for them. I have not seen a single expatriate living in Mumbai, and there are hundreds of them, venturing to drive in this huge city which boasts, among Indian cities, the most disciplined traffic culture!

If you keep yourself physically fit and accept a fair share of household chores there will be no creaks in the neck requiring an ugly collar, or shoulder and back pains, or frustrating physical ailments, or osteoporosis and you will be able to bend without clasping the small of the back. Some of my luxury inclined friends, who are averse to doing any household work which is relegated to domestic help, perennially complain of backaches and shoulder pains restricting their mobility and, generally speaking, are not in robust health. At sign of the slightest discomfort they run to the family physician and osteopath. I say to them do household chores and these minor physical intrusions will correct themselves naturally. Be patient. Nature has its own remedies.

Then there are those who cosset their lives with multi-coloured pills. Fifteen years ago on my transcontinental tour in the US on the AMTRAK from Washington D.C. to Ft. Pierce (Florida), I befriended a talkative and friendly, but not too healthy, American with a heart condition and some other ailments. He told me that to live he had to take 50+pills daily and to my horror he demonstrated this exercise by clutching a fistful of his daily quota and swallowed the same with gulps of water. Considering that I was then 75 he was very astonished when I told him my

daily intake was two pills—a multivitamin and a 50 mg. aspirin tablet.

Today there are millions who unknowingly could be risking their health and lives by over dosing themselves with multi-coloured pills some having serious side effects. Vitamin B6 taken by many women for pre menstrual tension, if taken in high doses, is believed to cause nerve damage. Vitamin A taken during pregnancy, without medical advice, is harmful to the unborn baby. There is some evidence that the popular vitamin C taken in high doses can even lead to the risk of cancer. There is a tendency to utilise vitamins as a substitute for an unhealthy life style or its excesses. Generally speaking, if you keep physically fit and your diet is healthy and balanced, there is no need to take vitamins unless they are medically prescribed particularly in old age to supplement vital deficiencies and give strength and vigour. Vitamin tablets are attractive and so easy and painless to swallow that to millions, particularly in western countries, they have become a part of their life style. It is reported that the consumption of drugs annually in USA is worth $ 1.10 trillion.

Referring to aspirin, it is known and established as a wonder drug preventing the clogging of arteries, transient ischemic attacks, strokes and colorectal cancer. It must be taken under medical supervision with the correct prescribed dose to avoid after effects such as internal bleeding. Aspirin is a life saver. It is estimated that aspirin/aspirin products account for about 20% of over the

counter drug sales in USA. The FDA of US has approved its uses for lower risk of death after heart attack, stroke and for relieving pain, fever and treatment of arthritis and lupus and has recommended its avoidance for asthma, severe kidney and liver diseases and bleeding disorders. For 50 years I have swallowed one 50 mg. tablet every night which may have been a contributory factor to my longevity.

To push ageing away by any means cosmetic surgery has boomed in recent years becoming a huge industry pandering particularly to the vanity of women. A variety of products are fiercely competing to cater to women's pursuit of the elusive fountain of youth. It is estimated that in UK 415,000 people have non-surgical cosmetic treatments and more than 75,000 cosmetic operations are performed each year with 90% patients being women. Middle aged women go for transplants for firming breasts having confidence in improved surgical techniques. Face lift surgery has become attractive for those who have crossed 60 and want to conceal their biological age. Frown lines, double chins, static wrinkles, sagging skins all go under the scalpel.

Women pay a fortune for what are called "cowboy" fixes which include quick flab jabs and even lunch time breast jobs with untested treatments. In non- surgical operations even hair dressers, dentists and beauticians have come on board to administer treatment without training which is accepted to save time and money. These facial remedies arc particularly targeting young women

with high pressure marketing who are induced to submit to surgery with attractive economic packages which are criticised by the Association of Plastic Surgeons as unethical.

The downside of failed facial surgery can be traumatic. In some cases, the surgery does little to improve the countenance while post surgery complications could be constant pain, broken blood vessels, drooping eyelids etc. requiring expensive regular surgical correction. In rare cases the surgery can even prove fatal. Reputed surgeons have warned against untested treatments but there is such a surge to conceal biological ageing that caution is thrown to the winds.

Speaking at a conference of British Association of Aesthetic Plastic Surgeons speakers condemned useless or dangerous products marketed through salons or internet and instances were given of breast enlargement procedure known as "celution" whereby fat or stem cells from the body are injected into the breasts. Fat melting treatments known as "Lipodissolve" or "Lipostabil" though banned are available on the internet. Anti-ageing injections of vitamins, herbs and minerals (known as mesotherapy) are all available without any scientific studies. It is very unfortunate that some persons for the sake of vanity are indulging in trying painful reversal of the process of ageing instead of accepting it gracefully.

Black and Asian women, keen to lighten the colour of their skin, are easy prey to high pressure publicity marketing facial creams and ointments which may look

effective but result in some cases in the skin becoming thin and dehydrated with the appearance of ugly boils and ulcers. There is a huge instant appealing market for products which promise to turn the complexion into fair and lovely and also fair and handsome. If the chemical contents used are harmful they may even lead to kidney and liver complications. It is imperative to read details of ingredients used and consult the family physician before embarking on any radical alteration of the skin in any form to prevent permanent scarring and damage. Be sure there is no short cut to restore youth and certainly not promote longevity.

It is interesting to read that Hollywood is now placing emphasis on natural looks. Casting editors are re-examining approach for the need for Botox, breast implants, nose jobs, specially treated lips, tautness of skin and other types of surgery which present a visibly artificial look. Soon days will come when starlets will not have to go for plastic surgery for casting.

In the rough and tumble of stress filled life in the modern age there are not many enduring pleasures left except a good night's undisturbed sleep. Getting up completely afresh is really one of life's untaxed little pleasure which we human beings have never adequately appreciated. How fervently we all look forward to getting into bed after a hard day at office or travel or partying.

The common perception is that a good night's sleep will go a long way to slow down the process of ageing whilst sleep deprivation will show up with dark circles under

the eyes, wrinkles, puffiness and an unhealthy looking pallor. I have previously referred to a recent study which indicates that to live for 100 years you need 10 hours of sleep. However, there is no definite accepted scientific study to support the conclusion that a good night's sleep promotes longevity. Baroness Margaret Thatcher, when she was Prime Minister for several years, is reputed to have slept for only 4 hours and she is now 84 though believed to be somewhat in frail health. On the other hand Calvin Coolidge, a former President of United States, slept 8 hours in the night and 3 in the afternoon .and lived till 63 only. Scientific thought is that sleep patterns have a lot to do with the genes of the family. In my 80s and even now when I am 90 I have been comfortable with 7 hours sleep in the night with a mandatory afternoon siesta of 30/45 minutes. If genes are important for longevity I must confess both my parents died at a relatively early age in their mid sixties.

I would like to add that there is a great virtue in the afternoon siesta. Even minimum of 30 minutes would be satisfactory, if time cannot be spared for a longer period of one hour. After you wake up, for the first 15 up to 30 minutes, you will be irritable, waspish and unpleasant whilst recovering your bearings, but after that you are ready to work till a late hour fresh and without fatigue and a woman particularly would have a look as fresh as Diana's visage. In India's largest industrial group where I worked the directors assembled to have a hearty lunch and then each repaired to his office suite to have a nap.

I have followed this practice all my adult life and I dare say I feel physically and mentally refreshed and active till midnight. I took up this habit after reading how Winston Churchill enjoyed his daily long afternoon siesta and then was wide awake till early morning, whilst the UK was fast asleep, calling all his cursing aids and generals during the last War at unearthly hours for discussion on military strategy and important affairs of state.

I cannot adequately emphasise that my longevity in the 92nd year is in good measure due to my addiction to an afternoon short siesta which eases all the physical and mental fatigue of the first 6 hours of the day. I use the word "addiction" which it is because when I get up after lunch I can barely open the newspaper before sleep takes over. Of course you can afford the siesta if you are retired and have no engagements to keep or are sufficiently senior in executive position to nap in your office suite. People living along the Mediterranean coast have made an art of the siesta, which extends to several hours between 1 to 4 pm with leisurely heavy lunch, when little business is conducted, and then they work hard till 8 to 9 pm.

As an individual I have never been bothered by ageing, though I am fully aware and have accepted that biological hallmarks denoting ageing such as skin lacking tautness, watery eyes, slight stooping, slowing of movement and partial hearing impairment have been my constant companions progressively increasing since I crossed 80. I give no more than a passing thought to this irreversible phenomenon and take them as par for the course. I went

bald early and began greying on the temples 30 years ago and was largely grey at 70. My ego was not punctured and I took no steps to dye my hair to look young and foolish when my face would betray my age. I deplore seeing dark dyed hair sitting on old looking faces of some of my friends. This is the normal fetish of women growing in age who are literally slaves to dyeing their hair an unnatural black to suppress their age and, if hospitalised, face the unacceptable mortifying prospect of looking horribly grey and white.

Ageing like mortality is ever present in our lives, admitting of no arguments, until the ongoing researches breach the frontiers of life. Attempts have been made in the laboratory to postpone death. South Korean scientists announced the development, which was subsequently reported to be fake and fabricated, of a method to clone human embryos and extract stem cells which would have revolutionised medical treatment by offering similar genetic matches. Had this research been true and successful the next step would have been to clone human beings in the laboratory which apparently is not far away with serious consequences to humanity.

Stem cell therapy where umbilical cord tissue from new born babies is injected into the body is becoming a big business for beauty doctors supposedly for its rejuvenating potential and satisfying the needs of women who want to look young. It is understood that Mr. George Bush, the former President of the United States, had expressed deep

concern and condemned stem cell therapy as "godless" vigorously opposing federal funding.

Nevertheless, recent advances in anti-ageing medicine may turn out to be beneficial and enable normally accepted life span to have a fresh look. Stem cell therapy is expected to act as a repair shop to grow new nerves, cure paralysis, detect cancer early, arrest the decline of vital organs and other developments which today lead to mortality much earlier. These advances could make it possible to live longer in a healthier condition and 100 could then be a relatively young age.

An American scientist has predicted that within as little as 20 years time, through nanotechnology and increased understanding of genes and computer technology, replacement of vital body organs will become common place and mankind's longevity will be limitless. In about 20 years time we will be able to re- programme our bodies and halt and reverse ageing. A fascinating world of nanobots will do work over a wide field thousands of time more effectively with immense possibilities.

Indeed if the final frontiers of life are breached it is possible that, in this century, life and death would be determined in the laboratory. What sort of people will then live and walk on earth? What effect will there be on the living space on the planet and the natural resources of food it provides? To meet the demand, would we have to supplement our staples of life, wheat, rice, grains, by production in the laboratory? With the increase in population would life on the planet be sustainable for

medical care, conservancy, housing, education etc.? Would religion die and God, as accepted in our consciousness today, cease to have any meaning? It is necessary to deeply ponder over these questions.

Chapter IV

**"Too much of anything is bad
But too much of whisky is rarely enough"**

Mark Twain

Dining Dieting and Quantitative Restrictions

I do not subscribe to Mark Twain's aphorism but it is undeniable that good food with wine is one of the elixir of life. Preparation of food, mixture of a myriad ingredients and finally its appetising presentation is a cultivated art which is unfortunately forgotten everywhere in the world, except in France and some western European and Asian countries, where eating well is still a cult.

Good food, if carefully prepared and digested, would give great pleasure through the whole course of life. However, the modern world is set on a junk food rampage popularised through seductive publicity and made available at affordable prices. To economise on

time, effort and money, it is so convenient and easy to pop into any of the thousands of fast food outlets selling hot dogs, hamburgers, fillets all encased in thick bread slices accompanied by fries, colas and fizzy waters. These have become the curse of life leading to mass obesity with severe health hazards.

There are more fat than hungry people in the world today with the unofficial count being more than a billion overweight and 800 million undernourished in World population estimated at 6 billions. In USA where junk food is believed to have originated, 30% of population or nearly 90 millions are reckoned to be obese on the basis of BMI (Body Mass Index calculated by dividing weight in kilograms by square of height in meters). According to the guidelines proposed by the World Health Organisation a BMI of up to 25 is healthy, more than 25 is overweight and over 30 obese. A report suggested that obesity rates in 2004 rose in all but one of the 50 states of the USA. Another survey indicated that one in four adults is clinically obese and nearly two-thirds are overweight.

Whilst the military abatement of violence and the noticeable decline in deaths in Iraq are a welcome sign the downside is the growing incidence of obesity amongst soldiers who now have a relatively easy life A dining table in the mess with its wide spread would pass away as a banquet but for the presence of soldiers in their fatigues. The Pentagon is worried since 5% or about 6000 are clinically obese if the total strength is 120000 approximately.

Diabetes, which is one of the off shoots of obesity, affects nearly 7 % of adults costing billions in health care and billions more in lost production. As a tourist I made two train journeys from New York to San Diego and from NY to Fort Pierce, Florida and I was astonished to see hugely obese people travelling on the trains and the tragedy was that several of them were young snacking on fries drowned with fizzy drinks. It is not surprising that, according to a recent survey by the American Institute of Cancer Research, obesity is the cause of 100,000 incidents of cancer in the US every year.

Scotland is the second fattest nation in the developed world after the US with alarmingly high levels of obesity in children which is considered to be horrific and a time bomb. Women particularly face serious health problems from being obese with 13 times more likelihood of developing Type 2 diabetes than those with normal weight.

A study of 10,000 people in England revealed that obesity level was increasing with children and adults continuing to get fatter. 30% of children are obese. In men, obesity had nearly doubled from about 13% in 1993 to 26% in 2005 with slightly lower rate of increase for women. This may have something to do with genes since recent findings indicate that DNA has a bearing on body size which makes it difficult to control food intake. Obesity continues unabated despite more people exercising and a boom in health food sales and use of gymnasiums to get fitter. It is estimated that 30,000 people died prematurely

every year from obesity related causes. What a preventable loss of lives?

Australia, world renown for athleticism and sporting achievements, is competing now with USA in battling the bulge. It is estimated that fat Aussies are costing their government nearly a billion dollars annually. They have been plumping for the "Total Well Being Diet" which is basically a low carbohydrate, high protein variation devised by Government scientists attached to Commonwealth Scientific and Research Organisation. This diet burst on the scene with eclectic effect with the book recording a sale of a million copies.

The new concept is that the quantity of fat in the diet is not that important but what matters is the intake of calories. Actually 200 gm. of red meat is recommended four times a week and the expected flak is deflected by the view that Australian meat is lean and nutritious compared to a low calorie diet which lacks adequate proteins and is nutritionally not enough. The diet has a structured approach giving a day by day healthy programme of weight reduction tailored to calorie requirements and, it is claimed, this could result in an estimated weight loss of 0.5 to 1 kg. per week, which is reckoned to be a sensible and healthy rate of weight loss. The diet asserts that it is a scientifically proven programme "challenging old conventions and theories".

All over the world people are becoming increasingly obese due to easy going life styles, more leisure seeking and the seductive bombing of consumers by aggressive

marketing of a variety of exotic foods and drinks available at affordable prices. Obesity has become such a problem that car manufacturers have even started enlarging sitting space. However, it is remarked that BMI per se should not be taken as the final verdict but an approximate indication as it does not take into account the build or muscularity of the person. What is important is the place where the visceral fat, otherwise accumulating dangerously in the abdomen, is distributed and located, particularly in women. It is said by some experts that a more accurate indication, is the waist size recommended to be 35 inches optimum in women and 40 in men. Like most other opinions this formula is also disputed.

Obesity is reckoned to be the second most important cause of death after tobacco. It is a great problem for the nations of the western world with incidence of consequential high cholesterol, skewed body image, diminishing self esteem, heart disease, arthritis, respiratory problems and osteoporosis, the last named being disastrous for women as they are more prone to it due to the fall in hormone level after menopause. Osteoporosis is a crippling bone disease causing fractures from the slightest fall. It causes ugly deformity with a pronounced curved back making it inconvenient to perform daily chores. It is estimated that 3 million people suffer from osteoporosis in the UK.

In 2005 there were 1.6 billion overweight adults in the world which number is estimated to increase to 2.3 billion by 2015. In some European countries more than 30% of

population is obese and more than 50% of all adults in Europe are classified as obese.

In "Super Size Me", Morgan Spurlock, in his box office documentary hit, demonstrated that he gained 25 pounds in a month eating fast food and in the process developed high cholesterol, signs of liver ailment, headaches, depression and sexual impotence. To reduce he went on the Detox diet, taking two months to shed 10 pounds and longer time to lose more, before returning to his previous athletic shape. This stunning observation should be noted by all those who mindlessly gorge themselves, particularly on holidays and sea cruises, believing that they would go on a diet later to shed excess weight. It is incredibly easy to gain weight and very exasperating to shed it.

I would say beware of structured diet schemes. They prey upon the fantasy and caprice of obese persons at great cost and possibly harmful effects offering a quick fix to get back to normal. They arrive promising the moon and some fade away in a short time and some last longer until results don't justify further existence or are replaced with more fanciful systems. Recently, scientists discovered that one of the most famous eating plans on sale could damage the heart. The findings raised concerns about blindly following structured diets. The company promoting the diet plan, which at one time had 3 millions hooked on it, is understood to have filed for bankruptcy in the USA and closed its operations in UK.

Fast food and soft drinks manufacturers are spending about $ 11 billions on advertising and, it must be said

to their credit that, responding to public outcry, they have been quick to react. Some of them have radically altered a part of their menus and servings by including salads and other health promoting foods with noticeable effect with the expert advice of nutritionists and dietary specialists. It will take some time before the damage is undone because burgers, fried chicken, fries and fizzy drinks continue to form a good proportion of servings. It must be remembered that a can of fizzy drink has 12 tea spoonfuls of sugar. Fast food outlets should voluntarily reduce the levels of salt (the silent killer), saturated fat and sugar.

It is no wonder these outlets are coming under increasing scrutiny of US Congress and the changes that are being made will take consumer heat off their backs. Following an agreement between major beverage distributors and anti-obesity advocates, millions of students in USA will no longer be able to buy non-diet sodas in public schools and instead only low fat milk and fruit juices will be available. Implementation will depend on the schools' willingness to change present arrangements. In UK, similar steps are being taken to vary afternoon lunch and snacks available in canteens. To fight obesity in India a proposal likely to be made into law is a blanket ban on junk food and colas in school and university canteens.

Business lunches and dinners on expense accounts, which are so trendy and a must in our high pressure corporate age, could be a disaster if not properly and

judicially handled. The vintage wines and lobsters, salmons and steaks with soufflés and crepe suzettes will undo all the abstinence that you have tortured yourself with in the preceding week. There is a way out though. Instead of approaching these feasts on your appointment list with an empty stomach, which some do so that they can gorge later, have a breakfast which is above the normal. At lunch avoid the aperitif and be abstemious with wine, which is a great seducer to make you eat substantial quantities of the sublime food. Be rational with the quantity of food consumed and try to avoid bread and butter at all costs. Be a mute spectator when the guys next to you begin to crunch the crusty bread before the first course is served (this is normally a French ritual). If you can help it, restrict your choice to fish and lean meats, with sufficient quantities of mildly dressed salads. It is not difficult to have fresh fruit sans crème instead of mouth watering sugared pastries. There is no restriction on the variety of food consumed and the only restraint is on the quantity.

I dine with society women, who are food fetishists and who to ease their malleable conscience are aficionados of one or other of the dietary systems but, over a period of time, I see little or no change in their body mass. They are the types whose weight loss is largely a mirage. I know women, who congratulate themselves on turning wholly vegetarian to reduce weight, but I am aghast watching them consume huge quantities of their dietary portions. When I remark, discretely and as mildly as possible, that this is not the right way I meet with stony uncomfortable

silence. They can well exclaim what Oscar Wilde said "I can resist everything except temptation".

What is the solution for obesity? The world is awash with different dietary methods which come highly acclaimed offering instant weight reduction and are adopted by millions with goodness knows what results. They play upon the vanity and caprice of people who basically have not taken care of themselves.

At any one time, there are available a proliferation of slimming drugs and new ones arrive on the market regularly. Amongst these are two obesity drugs one blocking the absorption of fat from the intestine, before it is digested, leading to weight loss and the other works on the brain making the person feel full and having no appetite to eat more. Although they claim they are well tested, they must be taken strictly under doctor's advice for protection against any life threatening after effects in the process of losing weight. It is gathered that researchers are working on developing a chewing gum that will curb appetite with a hunger- suppressing hormone.

Also, a whole range of medical and surgical treatments are available to reduce weight. There are weight reducing surgeons who perform laparoscopic gastric bending, sleeve gastrectomy, gastric bye- pass and reconstructive surgeons (plastic) catering to liposuction, abdominoplasty and tummy tucks. It is claimed that it is possible to lose 50 % of excess weight after gastric binding. Latest examples of those who benefited from this type of surgery are a former Argentine football star, who is reputed to have

lost nearly 27 kg. and a famous pop star who lost 18 kg. There is no reason to doubt these claims but this does not mean one should blindly opt for this type of surgical intervention without the advice and recommendation of the family physician.

In rare cases the downside can be disastrous. There is the unfortunate report of the wife of the President of an African country who died of complications following cosmetic surgery to reduce body fat. Very recently it is reported that former Miss Argentina in her prime lost her life after going under the knife for firming her buttocks. The procedure involved injections which led to acute respiratory problems leading to embolism and death. Surgical reduction of body fat could be dangerous and, it is claimed, that one in ten patients suffer from post operative complications leading possibly to fatal results. It would be advisable always to assess consequences and after effects before embarking on serious surgical procedures.

Now I come to the most important recommendation I would like to make on controlling bodyweight. My theory of keeping weight and BMI in check, provided you are already not obese beyond redemption, is simple and effective from personal experience and is very agreeable. Avoid greasy preparations and eat large portions of vegetables, eat everything including rice, potatoes, meat and, with effective quantity control, even lobster, mildly sugared pastries and exotically prepared foods. Impose on yourself no dietary restriction except, and this is very

important, get up from the table when you are feeling 25% hungry and avoid snacking between meals.

This is not very difficult to judge or estimate, and can be very simple to put into practice, if you are honest to yourself and feel you can wallop more and stop at that level. Follow this recommendation religiously and it will do wonders to your weight control and, at the same time, give you immense pleasure at being able to eat different varieties of delectable foods. This will allow persons who are mildly obese to bring down their weight to less than the obesity level. I feel convinced that no amount of walking, swimming or gym. work are weight reducing and the only way is to reduce the quantity of food intake.

For those who are highly obese the only recourse is to significantly cut down on quantitative intake of food but with careful care and constant watch that the other peril of *anorexia* and *bulimia nervosa* are not reached which will be difficult to shake off resulting in complete loss of appetite. I discourage the total skipping of meals which is a growing obsession and is fashionable amongst youngsters to maintain their body shape. Ladies who have gone to the other extreme of dieting are known to develop bulimia and look emaciated and are finding it extremely difficult to regain body weight.

What more does one want to enjoy all the delights of good food but accompanied by self imposed restraint. I repeat eat everything but get up 25% hungry when you feel you want and can eat more very easily. You will be

comfortable, not bloated, interesting at a party and not behave as a social moron, feeling drowsy, wanting to go home to hit the bed instead of being convivial and a bright conversationalist. In the night, you will not begin to snore the moment you go under the sheet, but will be more solicitous of the tenderness which your partner is anxiously expecting.

There will be no harmful effects on your bodily functions and, once you become used to this discipline, there will be no adverse effect on your normal physical activity. I am not saying you should disregard all the constructive talk of proteins, carbohydrates, fats and nutritional foods but do not make it as article of faith. If I am active and keeping busy in my 92nd year blessed with unfailing memory of events of the last 70 years, so can you be once you cross 60, enjoying all the culinary and other delights which life offers.

By choice there need not be over indulgence in anything you eat—for example you cannot just eat a two pound steak and nothing else. Do certainly eat lean tenderloin accompanied by vegetables and other foods. Similarly you are not breaking any secret code by eating lobsters or caviar or salmon in reasonable quantities as a gourmet and not as a *gourmand*.

For women losing weight, even moderately, will not only act as an aphrodisiac but with a better and more attractive physique will lead to a satisfying and more fulfilling sex life. In course of time stomach capacity will be reduced and inclination to eat will be less and less

without in any way affecting physical activity, alertness and sprightliness. Try this simple method and see what a world of difference it makes to life.

Recently, it was reported that Dr. Steven Hawk of Brigham Young University in Provo, Utah, USA dealing with what he calls "intuitive eating" declared, after a pilot study, that there is no need to diet, and intuitive eaters "recognise what our body wants and then regulate how much we eat based on hunger and satiety." It is mentioned that Asians are primarily intuitive eaters—they eat when hungry and stop when full and that Asians have a healthier relationship with food, far fewer eating disorders and less obesity. The view is also expressed that "diets and dieting often fail to result in long-term weight loss, largely because food restriction works against human biology, is not sustainable, and may lead to negative outcome such as weight recycling, altered body composition, increased fat storage, decreased metabolism and eating disorders".

What I have recommended-- getting up from the table when you feel you are 25 % hungry-- is somewhat similar and my view is supported by practising this habit all through my life maintaining my body weight at a healthy BMI.

There is a food programme known as "calorie restriction" (CR) which, in its basics, claims that by reducing the calorie intake to 40% of 2500 recommended by the British Nutrition Foundation, the ageing process can be slowed down. This programme is based on the finding that, rats fed on a restricted calorie regime, lived up

to 50% longer than those who were not subjected to this restriction. The discovery reported to be based on work done in the Biology Department of Cornell University is yet to be scientifically established whether it will work on humans without serious side effects due to deficiency in vital nutrients. Very simply it is claimed a low calorie diet will slow down the biological process of ageing. A word of caution which is not related to obesity or weight control. Be careful barbecue preparations, popular in the summer, have been identified as carrying carcinogens normally present in the burnt part of portions grilled by charcoal.

Do certain foods have aphrodisiac qualities? It is the general belief that bananas, basil, carrots, ginger, chocolates, garlic, oysters, etc. enhance sexual prowess similar to consuming preparations made from rhinoceros horns and testicles of tigers (never to be encouraged to protect these magnificent but vanishing species of wild life). However, the US Food and Drug Administration have put an official damper by declaring that the sexual powers in food items essentially belong to folk lore. If the FDA finding is universally known and accepted it would be a shot in the arm essentially for the preservation of the world's wild life.

A leading London daily listed the following top foods for longevity, Cabbage, kale, broccoli, sprouts (contain Indole-3-Carbinol) which help to fight lung and breast cancer Blueberries contain resveratrol found in grapes and red wine—powerful in retarding ageing and can even reverse failing memory Nuts—two servings of 8

gm. a week lower risk of heart attack and almonds and walnuts lower cholesterol Tomatoes—10 servings of sauce or tomatoes a week reduces risk of prostate cancer

Garlic—prolongs cancer survival time in animals by about 5 % which in humans might add about 4 years

Oily fish contains high levels of omega-3 fatty acids which protect the heart

Let me touch briefly on garlic, the wonder drug. It's therapeutic quality cannot be under estimated. Garlic contains vitamins B and C, amino acids and minerals, purifies blood, prevents blood clotting and bad cholesterol.

It can assist weight loss by burning fat through stimulation of adrenalin. It has anti-fungus, anti-viral, anti-bacterial properties. Garlic's detoxifying properties could assist in improving memory and reducing risk of blood pressure in pregnancy.

Garlic is an important ingredient in French cuisine and the French are the world's largest consumer at an annual average of 800 gm. per capita. King Henry IV, the 16th century monarch, who was known to be a successful philanderer, was reputed to owe his conquests to consuming garlic at breakfast. But with all its miraculous properties how is one to neutralise the highly pungent odour it produces on chopping and, unless it is eaten raw, its potency is somewhat diminished. It is an ideal ingredient for a bachelor with no female entanglement.

Eggs, which are being roundly condemned as high in cholesterol and difficult to digest, are ideal for not only

breakfast but for lunch and dinner providing proteins, minerals including iron and zinc, vitamins and are low in sodium. A single egg, which contains about 80 calories and 5 gm.of fat, is highly nutritious. It is an indispensable item of food. The yolk provides 13 essential nutrients and the white contains albumen with no fat. Eggs are also rich in iodine. Some research suggests they can also help in reducing weight. The famous English breakfast of two eggs accompanied by meats, cereals, jam, butter, fruits and beverage of choice has much to commend itself provided the egg quantity is reduced to one and the helpings of bacon, ham and sausages are reasonable.

Studies have shown that reduced intake of salt lowers the blood pressure and incidence of heart disease and strokes. Despite increasing awareness in the food processing industry about its harmful effects, there is still too much addition of salt, and health experts have not ceased to issue alerts that food should not be peppered on the table with extra salt. It has been identified that, as against the maximum safe consumption level of 6 gm a day, the average adult consumes 9 to10 gm.and, according to researchers, shaving just 3gm.off the daily intake would prevent 92000 deaths in the US and save $24 billion in health costs on treating tens of thousands of patients suffering from strokes and heart attacks.

For daily function of nerves and muscles of the human body and also to regulate fluids, we require just 1 gm., which is the barest minimum biological requirement, against 9 gm. consumed today. Most adults, consuming

packaged foods, have a daily average intake of 10 gm. and for meat consumers this mounts up to the high risk figure of 15 gm. For children, a bag of chips is the worst culprit with a tag of 1 gm. and how many are consumed daily is anybody's guess. A slice of bread contains 0.50 gm. and a bowl of corn flakes adds 1gm. Alarmed at the growing salt menace, doctors are advising giving up chips and reducing consumption of bread, ham, bacon and pizza. Salt manufacturers are alarmed at the adverse propaganda against salt and reject the accusation that "the path to a hospital bed is sprinkled with salt". The healthy solution would be to ban salt from the dining table and thus avoid extra addition above what is already added during food preparation.

New York is in the forefront of changing harmful dietary habits. Following the ban on smoking in all closed areas and introducing the recent ban on trans fats in restaurants, officials have recognised the harmful effects of excessive salt consumption which is a major health problem. Several health organisations have joined to implement what is called the National Salt Reduction Initiative to target the average American's salt consumption and reduce it by 20% in 5 years since they eat twice as much as they need to for better health. Manufacturers are called upon to reduce salt gradually in preparation so that it is not noticeable.

Let me write briefly about spices which not only bring exotic taste to food but have medicinal properties. I have already described the virtues of garlic. Coriander seeds

having anti- inflammatory properties are being studied for cholesterol reduction, turmeric is being researched for its potential to prevent cancer, chillies which are used extensively by Indians in food preparation have a range of health benefits like relief from pain, reducing congestion, preventing stomach ulcers and even weight loss. Ginger's anti-inflammatory properties is nature's remedy for heart burns, migraine, colds, flu and menstrual cramps and is also being researched as treatment for ovarian and colon cancer.

What should be the quantity of food to be eaten at breakfast, lunch and dinner? I have already expressed in detail the great virtue of getting up from the table when feeling 25 % hungry. I don't subscribe to the saying "breakfast like a king, lunch like a prince, dine like a pauper." To the best of my knowledge, the practice in continental Europe is to have a light breakfast of croissant and coffee followed by a good lunch with wines and then by a light supper which usually consists of soup, cheese, pastry and fruits.

In Mediterranean countries, lunch is the real meal of the day followed by a siesta. The body's capability of digesting food is best during the day and a heavy dinner is not advisable. Much depends not only on individual habits but also on snacking and nibbling on tit bits between meals which dulls the appetite and should be avoided. It is worth while to bear all this in mind to promote long enjoyable life with good health.

Is there anything substantial in the belief that active gymnasium work out is weight reducing? I have my sincere doubts. It is very fashionable and is a welcome way to keeping the body fit and well toned and, with special exercises, develop muscle strength, posture and shape but, unless it is combined with quantitative restrictions on food, I doubt whether gym. work per se is weight reducing. When I ask obese friends to reduce, the pat reply comes "I go to the gym. daily" as if that is a cure for obesity. Do not rely solely on gym.work for weight reduction.

Walking falls in the same category. It is said that 40 km. of power walking with sweating may reduce weight by one kilo (I have dealt separately the great need to walk for fitness and good health). Spas which are so fashionable in western countries are not in any noticeable way weight reducing though they are good for relaxation and toning when accompanied by a massage. The present fad is ayurvedic massage with ointment prepared from Indian herbs for which the discerning rich visit India, particularly the south. All these fads can assist in weight reduction provided they are accompanied with quantitative restrictions on food.

I would now like to refer to nature's great benefaction, without any cost if judicially used, which is vitamin D available in plenty from the warmth of the sun. It is an essential nutrient by chemical reaction when ultra violet rays fall on the body. If UV rays are not carefully controlled they could lead to disastrous consequences causing skin

cancer. Ultra violet radiation is the biggest cause of skin damage and cancer. Lying in the sun on beaches, on the special spas created on terraces of high rise boutique hotels and also in tanning salons for hours to ensure a nice copper tan, even protected by various creams available in the market, is most inadvisable. When sun bathing, protection from the shade of an umbrella or a tree, if prolonged, is at least 50% lethal.

Though they are very attractive to look at I am appalled to see beautiful women with their copper tan bodies lying exposed for hours on the French Riviera, unmindful of the risk of skin cancer associated with unbridled exposure to the UV rays. I knew a lady whose fad was to take daily the tropical harsh sun for hours with so called sun cream protection. She had an enviable tan and did not die of cancer of the skin but she looked haggard and aged much beyond her age with conspicuous ugly wrinkles on face and neck.

Vitamin D will ward off influenza, reduce risk of osteoporosis, rickets, bowel cancer, diabetes, dementia etc. Foods which are rich in vitamin D are oily fish, eggs and breakfast cereals. A recent study on ageing has reported that high vitamin D levels leads to greater mental agility in men aged 40 to 80.

I think it would be worth while to relate below my daily diet

Morning (about 0730 hours)

Two cups of tea with one slice of buttered toast before 2 km. walk

Breakfast (about 1000 hours)

>   Small bowl of corn flakes with half tea spoon of sugar and dash of milk or cut of any French/Swiss cheese on one unbuttered toast, slice of papaya or melon and one wine glass of orange juice

Lunch (about 1330 hours)

>   One course generally of Indian ethnic non-vegetarian food including occasionally rice and dessert

Dinner (about 2100 hours)

>   One light course of Indian ethnic non-vegetarian food with seasonal salads and dessert
>
>   Sometimes I treat myself to a glass of white or red wine and cognac
>
>   No aperitif or hard liquor (except on social occasion)
>
>   No second serving
>
>   No supper
>
>   No snacking between lunch and dinner
>
>   No pre-lunch application of butter on bread
>
>   No sprinkling of salt
>
>   I am not fond of caviar but enjoy lobster and smoked salmon.

My most important approach towards food is to get up from the table when I feel I am 25% hungry.

I feel despondent that in the light of millions in India going to sleep without a square meal my food intake, though normal for a middle income individual, would be equivalent to sitting at a banquet. I am overcome with remorse but I am helpless. I want the reader to bear with

me when I write that I can not stem the onslaught of the
ocean with a shovel in my hand!!

Chapter V

"Tis not a year or two shows us a man:
They are all but stomachs, and we all but food;
They eat us hungerly, and when they are full,
They belch us."

Emilia in *Othello*

Sex Marriage and Longevity

"Sex is one of the nine reasons for reincarnation—the other eight are unimportant" Henry Miller. It is unarguable that good food and the enjoyment of sex are the primordial instincts of mankind and equally very important for longevity. You eat to live well, you have sex to fulfil your life. Good sex is a cherished event in life and has to be approached with finesse and consummated with joy. Emotions and mood must meet to have any sexual meaning unless it is instant sex at first sight made famous by a well known tennis star. Then there is the other end of sex which is maniacal as the wife of a football star of yester

year confessed in her autobiography that her husband wanted sex 10 times a day and she added that it was better to succumb than be beaten up (later denied).

Without sex, life is as barren as the sands of Sahara and withers like a plant without water. Life without sex is acutely frustrating and is no recommendation for a long and healthy life. Lack of sex leads to all kinds of mood disorders and secondary ailments. Headaches, backaches, imaginary illnesses, abnormal behaviour, choleric temper all become a part of the sexually deprived person.

Whether you are married or single and young or old, sex truly is never out of your mind. The effect of sex on mind, body, good health and longevity, indulged in even when well past 60, especially with one you are fond of, can only be described as ethereal. There is nothing more satisfying and even gourmet food is secondary. Enjoyment of sex is not the exclusive preserve of youth and, if you are fit, reasonably attractive, posses a charming disposition and have an agreeable partner, believe me, there will be no erectile problem even in early 80s. I have no qualms in saying that I have indulged in the most enjoyable sex until I was well into my 80s. It has acted as an aphrodisiac to my longevity.

If you are in your 60s, do not feel despondent and carry the belief that you have ceased to be potent. There is nothing unusual in erotic thoughts when coming into visual contact or close proximity to an attractive female. Physical stimulation and foreplay between partners well into their 60s will leave them in utter amazement. It is

quite possible that men in their 60s, having lost their youthful skin sensitivity, may be able to last sufficiently longer to give satisfactory orgasm to the partner.

It is said that sex, as it involves physical and emotional effort, is risky and not safe for an ageing body. Moderate sexual activity (not with a teenager), at reasonable intervals, would be emotionally very satisfactory, particularly with an intimate partner. Nevertheless, there are age related frequency limits to sexual enjoyment, and it is difficult to accept the statement made a few years ago by India's celebrated painter, who is now about 93, that the most satisfying sexual time of his life had just begun!

Indian media recently reported that an 88 year old Indian farmer living in the sand dunes of Rajasthan, one of the Indian states, had become the proud father of a baby boy. His wife, 43 years old, delivered twins of whom one was still born. The story is that his two previous wives, not being able to give him a son, which is very important in India, actually encouraged him to take another wife. He does not smoke or drink, eats very simple food, as all farmers do, enjoys sex daily, glorifying it for good health, and says the best time to indulge in it is between 2 and 4 AM !

Recently the coaching management of the Indian cricket team presented the players with a vision document (later denied) encouraging them to improve their on the pitch performance by having sex the previous night and a leading sexologist supporting this added that this can lead to fantastic performance in the outdoor sport. The thinking

is that sex increases the levels of testosterone leading to greater strength, aggression and competitiveness. This is quite a reversal of the thinking when players on long tours were discouraged to have "romps" until lately when wives and girl friends (wags) are being allowed to join on long tours. The Indian coach has been lauded and some other teams in a light hearted manner have welcomed him to join their coaching management.

Nevertheless, as a man advances in age, he need not behave like Casanova (1725-1798), the Italian adventurer prince famous for his romantic escapades in 18th century libertine European society who charmed his way through life seducing women; nor like Marquis de Sade (1740-1814), whose erotic writings and perverse sexual preferences, in which prostitutes played an important part, gave rise to the term "sadism".

On the subject of marriage what you are about to read may seem heretical but I pray it should be read dispassionately. Let me be very clear I am not a critique of the institution of marriage which is as old as the hills. What is important is that marriage must endure and should be made to play an integral part in promoting longevity. As long as society requires legitimacy to be attached to children and, as long as illegitimate children face social stigma as in India but not so in developed countries, the institution of marriage will survive. Also, it may be that one of the important virtues of marriage which gives it legitimacy is the exchange of genes. Being a happily married man for 10 years I know how marriage

can brighten life, if only it is properly nurtured, with all the pleasures of physical and mental bonding.

For a long happy marriage well into 60s and beyond, it would be advisable for the man and the woman to have a healthy difference in age at the time of marriage, which I would say should be ideally at least 5 years, with the woman being younger. It is natural to fall in love at an early age, but the consequences of contracting marriage at an early age, when you are just out of your teens, and with slight difference in age, would be appalling as you grow older. Women in their twenties beware that men are much quicker on the draw than them in proposing as romantic mood races in their minds like fire as compared to women who are wisely calculating with their feet firmly on the ground. Assess the proposal and contemplate it with "due diligence" to avoid bitter disappointment later. May be all this is theoretical for a mature person but blurting out "I love you" is so natural in an excited moment when you are young that the words come out like a pistol shot mindless of future consequences.

Why am I suggesting an age difference? As you reach 40s, the physiological difference in looks and physique begin to be apparent. A woman in her 40s weighed down by child bearing, raising a family, looking after the home and all its domestic chores begins to show the scars of ageing. Comparatively, a man in his 40s is emerging into his prime in looks, bearing, presence and personality. With every year added after 40, the woman is biologically and visibly going over the hills developing sagging skin,

withered complexion, ungainly weight which would be in marked contrast to her husband if they are more or less of the same age.

There are rare exceptions of women being attractive to men when they are in their 40s and 50s and, if they are, they are usually adorned with facial uplift and have kept themselves physically attractive. But a man, at this age, is drawing attention and envy if he is fit, in good condition, mentally alert and successful in life. Unarguably many women in their 20s will confess how attracted they are to men even in their 40s and above mainly for manliness, maturity and sexual attraction. Some go for security offered by a successful man and some others tag themselves with a celebrated doctor, scientist, actor or author.

With a minimum 5 years age difference, a woman could always feel safe, and will have a much better chance of protecting her marriage from prying eyes, and keep engaged her man's attention and continued interest in later years. As they grow older, men are attracted undeniably to much younger women not necessarily with any Lolita complex or to collect trophies but due to genuine physical attraction. If the wife wants her man to "stop looking", she must ensure that she is youthful looking, not plump and a dowdy baggage. This is very important, because the man will have so many opportunities to meet and get attracted to younger women at his work place, in business conferences, cocktails and business tours. Remember out there is a jungle and mine field of prowling single women, single mothers and women frustrated in marriage always

on the look out to snare men away. Everything will be hunky dory when young, but the true revelation of lack of adequate disparity in age will strike, when the woman reaches 40 and shows advancing age.

I may sound unusual and swimming against the tide if I express the view, honestly believing, that sleeping in king size beds by married couples or by live-in partners, with about 8 hours daily exposure and intimacy, could be the cause for the early disappearance of the shine in sexual relationship due to the loss of the all important *mystique* of the female body in the mind of the male partner and vice versa. Unfortunately, this sharing is the *sine qua non* of marriage, which is dictated in our age by scarce accommodation and also because social norms require that married couples sleep in the same bed, if for nothing than at least for bonding, however disagreeable either of them has become, having developed unacceptable habits over a period of time like snoring, farting, selfishly keeping the light on, rattling away on the lap top etc. The partner who is short changed would be reminiscing nostalgically of the pre-marriage outings when being solicitous to the needs and comforts of each other was the prime consideration. No matter how broad minded we are, it is unfortunate, that sleeping apart gives wrong signals of irreconcilable differences or a rift in marriage.

Coming out of the bath wrapped around in a towel with dangling breasts, sitting before the mirror in inner garments to complete the facials and going through the motions of dressing, all in the presence of the husband, are

a sure disaster for the continuation of passion and freshness in sexual relationship. Sexual passion is a priceless invisible mystique which has to be nurtured by least exposure. Do not make female nudity common place. It is very exciting and passionate when it remains a novelty and rare to behold but with too much exposure it becomes just passé. A man clothed is handsome; a woman partially clothed is divine. What is unseen in a female looks mysterious and best. Queen Victoria is reputed to have said "An ugly body is a very nasty object—the prettiest is frightful when undressed."

The mystique of the female body, which you were dying to unravel whilst courting with roses, is gone and is no more. That same mystique relating to the physical charms of a woman, the velvety Helen- like smoothness of her skin, her body's natural odour, the perfumed sensitive zones, the hairy tufts, the bewitching smile, have all become prosaic, if not dead. It is not a slow death. It comes like a thunderclap and when it dawns suddenly the touch of the partner becomes just symbolic devoid of any sexual arousal. Those days looking into each other's eyes with passion and love are never going to return.

This is why, after a few months of physical bonding, with all conceivable *Kama Sutra* (the ultimate manual on sex by Vatsyayana dating back to 300 AD) postures are exploited and enjoyed, there is the chilling response in the night in bed with one partner reading and the other snoring or the wife seething for sex but the husband is in oblivion. Emilia's cry in Othello is so prescient and true to

life. This could only happen with physical estrangement due to constant exposure. What is left is the obligatory civility of saying "good night" and that too many times grudgingly. The "iron curtain" of sexual desire and passion is irretrievably drawn. The dreaded stark bedroom boredom has set in.

Once the mystique is lost no matter what you do you can never bring back the good old times of candle lit dinners, walks in the parks and on the river bank, a visit to the opera or concert sitting rubbing shoulders for which you so assiduously looked forward to. The joy and careful selection of flowers for her and her sublime radiance when receiving them are just fond memories of the past. After some years, even selection of flowers for her on her birthday becomes a ritual best left to the secretary or florist!

The female you thought was so curvaceous and luscious, whose very presence and natural body odour put you into an erectile mode whilst courting, is no longer able to arouse your testosterone. Neither is able to say the magical words "I love you" and, if this is somehow belched out of the system, it would be a dishonest action devoid of any meaning or significance. During courtship, the male particularly is hungry to devour physically the woman he loves and waits for an opportunity to do so but when love has become a stranger each partner will make every attempt to avoid intimacy which has become chilling. Neither a transatlantic voyage nor a week in Bermuda is going to bring back the mystique and, in fact,

what would be uppermost in their minds would be how quickly the pretences would come to an end.

You can nostalgically recall that, once upon a time, the touch of entwined fingers whilst walking or looking into each other's eyes used to send a magnetic quiver of profound emotional significance leading to instant arousal and a sudden outflow of chemistry. Then as Shakespeare wrote "young men's love lies not in their hearts but in their eyes". Both of you were dripping wet in each other's company. When courting going out to dine was a special intensely looked forward occasion. Whatever was the level of conversation it was deemed interesting and free flowing, but now it is a chore with hardly a word exchanged. When love and passion are no more, whilst going home, holding fingers is like holding strings.

I am not wrong in writing that the mystique or the physical attraction of the human body is all important in binding partners. I question how is it that a stunning, beautiful wife for whom men would be prepared to give an arm and a leg has become sour to her husband and is on the divorce block unless it is because she has lost her mystique in his eyes. Men are prepared to give a fortune in settlement just to get rid of the partner no matter how attractive and beautiful she is. An insurance magnate is reputed to have paid his wife £48 million in divorce settlement in UK. A Russian oligarch is reputed to have paid £155 million. Divorces certainly don't come cheap and what price men put to secure them, in most cases to be free to be with another woman, is simply unimaginable.

Recent divorce decisions in UK are so favourable for the wife receiving not only a good part of present wealth but also a share of future earnings that divorce lawyers are advising clients to avoid walking the altar altogether.

A time comes when the partners and more often the man will be yearning for "space" to do something different, meet his buddies, visit a local, play golf or go fishing or to a ball game. Listening to mutual conversation, which was so animated and interesting when courting, becomes a drag. I am reminded of a cartoon which appeared in the satirical magazine "Punch" (1878) of a honeymooning couple sitting on the beach with the wife on a rock and husband at her feet in the sand. After having exhausted all topics of conversation and finding little interesting in each other's company, Angelina the wife, suppressing an inclination to yawn, exclaims "How nice it would be if some friend were to turn up, wouldn't it Edwin" to which Edwin, after yawning elaborately, replies "yes, or even an enemy"!

It is unarguable that the happiest romantic period in a person's life are the days of courting, which should be nourished and prolonged as long as possible. It is the time when everything is conspiring to be fresh like the morning dew and smells of roses. You are looking forward to be together to walk to drink to eat to converse to look into each other's eyes to hold hands with the chemistry flowing and the world be damned. I see in the searing and scorching afternoon heat of summer in Mumbai young couples in love sitting arms entwined on

the marina getting roasted and totally unmindful of the busy populated world around them which they would never dream of doing after marriage. A question may be asked why does everything ebb and what was expected to be eternal romance becomes common place and prosaic on getting married or living as partners and gradually vanishes until it is dead.

It is revealed that Chopin told his wife Lita Grey, who was pregnant with his child, to jump in front of a train. Recently, the estranged wife of a famous pop star deposed in court that when she was nursing the new born her husband shouted at her "those breasts are mine". These may be extreme cases of maniacal disposition which demonstrate in a way what happens to marriages, if they are not sufficiently and constantly kept in bloom, without losing the body's mystique.

I am not impressed to hear that a very important part of married life is companionship which may be a substitute but not an exciting one. Of course companionship does play a significant part in many marriages so does sex unless it is denied due to involuntary incapacity of either partner. Nevertheless in many marriages when there is physical ability, denial of sex raises dangerous alternatives including extra marital affairs. In quite a number of marriages and amongst live-in partners, inability to get along, irreconcilable differences, continuous and inconclusive petty arguments, incompatibility all unarguably flow when sex life becomes barren.

Generally speaking women of all ages are satisfied with their sex lives and for many their vision does not range beyond their husbands or partners. For the men it is a different ball game and they are prone to straying and to satisfy their conscience they rationalise by believing rightly or wrongly that they are dissatisfied in their sexual life or more crassly put they want a new toy something fresh before their middle age runs out.

Except in very rare cases all marriages, including of so called legendary people, have faced some degree of turbulence during their life span. This may arise partly due to husbands deeply involved in their political career or in revolutionary fight for freedom causing unavoidable separation from wives who mostly lump it and rarely revolt.

Are marriages generally successful? They must be otherwise why should people get married spending a phenomenal sum, which it is gathered costs about £27000 on an average in UK and the fact that the institution of marriage is the accepted ritual of our lives. A well known New York realtor correctly remarked "Marriage is greatest institution in the world when you get it right". It is said that in USA $ 80 billion (£50 billion) is spent annually on weddings and for UK the estimate for 2006 was £23 billion ($37 billion) even though 4 in 10 will end up in heart breaking or sordid divorce or separation. Queen Elisabeth II, who celebrated her 60th wedding anniversary in November 2007, is reputed to have despatched 280,000 telegrams to couples in the UK and the Commonwealth

who had completed 60 years of marriage. We take it for granted that all these fortunate couples are still happily married.

There is the rare case reported some years ago of a farmer couple from China's Guangxi province married for 83 years. The husband is 101, the wife 100. He does not smoke but drinks a small quantity of rice wine, is a vegetarian, eats potatoes to help digest food and ginger to keep away colds. Charles Darwin was married to the same woman for 43 years, loved children, dogs and plants, particularly orchids, and when not researching or writing reclined comfortably spending his time smoking.

If the high and unacceptable divorce rate in the western world is anything to go by then it is arguable whether marriages are the ideal solution for happy longevity. With divorce rate inexorably rising, invariably due to a third person entering the marriage equation, is it time to reflect whether keeping with changing times the marriage vow "Until death do us part" should not be changed to "Till three becomes a crowd". When marriages break down, the pre-divorce period of hostility at home with its traumatic effect on children, legal formalities for division of the estate, the costs involved, post divorce trauma of one of the partners suddenly not having a home to live, and most importantly, what to do with children and the impact on them, would be a disastrous period in the lives of the parents affecting their longevity.

As compared to the husband, the ordeal for the wife of a broken marriage is highly traumatic both physically

and emotionally which is not eased even by taking a new partner. Recently the divorced wife of one of the most celebrated personality of the last century is reputed to have confessed that the desolation caused by her broken marriage has led to relentless pain at being abandoned and feeling alone which apparently the millions of pounds obtained in divorce settlement had in no way helped to mitigate.

Marriage is not something of an event in life once contracted to be left to nurture itself and succeed on its own. It is a partnership of love and emotion involving a tremendous amount of compromise and understanding which are the buzz words. Living together both partners would suddenly face the fact that each of them is so different in attitude, behaviour, standards of tidiness, interest in games, use of leisure time and emotional responses all uncomfortably different from what was experienced during the courting period. Individualism and its assertion in marriage without compromise would be a disaster.

In contemporary times with increasing female empowerment and ambition to scale to career heights, the marriage equation is getting increasingly blurred. Will the husband be satisfied if the wife career bound continues to delay rearing a family and instead of serving warm roast beef cooked to his liking gives him a cold sandwich which she grabs on the way home? Would he be able to complain if the comforts and life style enjoyed by him are substantially due to her earnings and what if she brings

work home and rattles away on her lap top in the night? Forbes magazine's Michael Noer's advice to men is worth quoting "marry pretty women or ugly ones, short ones or tall ones, blondes or brunettes, just whatever you do don't marry a woman with a career"!

Unarguably, infidelity is the most common cause for divorce. Except in cases where the married couple voluntarily slides along and keeps the facade of marriage going for the sake of young children or not to harm the political ambition or status of the husband, there is zero tolerance in marriage for *la ménage à trois* or as a famous Princess once said "three is a crowd". Are men more unfaithful than women? This is debatable. On the face of it men appear to be more promiscuous but this is because they are not smart enough to cover their philandering tracks or shall we say women are smarter than men and if they are promiscuous they know how to cover their tracks.

Men think they are clever in obliterating their trail of infidelity but they drop clues unintentionally like confetti. Recently, the most celebrated sports icon of the century reputed to be worth $500 million + married ostensibly happily for 5 years with two infants was allegedly found to have been unfaithful having a string of mistresses who came out of the wood work. He thought he was smart in covering his steps but when the time came it seemed he had left a gushing trail. The media was unforgiving and he is valiantly trying to save his marriage. His wife is a well brought up beautiful blonde being the daughter of a

cabinet minister of a European country attractive enough to draw appreciative attention of any man. What went wrong? Was it the loss of *mystique* I have written about or is he kind of sexual athlete requiring counselling?

Is extra marital sex necessary for successful men to achieve greater career successes? Is this a way out to release their pent up emotions and testosterones and fulfil their lives? It appears to be so with power sex acting as a stimulant for which men have risked their highly successful business and political careers and high profile marriages at substantial financial cost.

Some of the Presidents of USA and British Prime Ministers, well known in history for their marital infidelity, were always careful to keep their philandering under wraps to ensure there was no blotch on their political careers. Lately a French President's long extra marital affair was only revealed publicly when the mistress appeared with the grown up love child of all places at his funeral. King Edward VII, allegedly well known for his jousts with women, had made Paris and Biarritz his favourite jaunts and, in fact, the well known 5 star Hotel Prince des Galles in Paris is supposedly named after him. There is the story that once when the British cabinet requested him to return to London for discussion on a very important matter of state he declined as he could not leave Biarritz and invited the whole cabinet to come to Biarritz instead!

Men alone are not the unfaithful scoundrels. A British lady manor born cuckolded her husband who was the

British Prime Minister for several years, and not that the husband was blissfully unaware. Well Frenchmen are a case apart where women are concerned. It is said, and I cannot vouch for the belief, that a Frenchman has no status in Paris without a mistress. When you are married must you avoid admiring attractive women? There is a saying that "a woman is as old as she looks and a man is old the moment he stops looking". Franz Kafka truly said "anyone who keeps the ability to see beauty never grows old."

How does one keep marriage alive and vibrant? There is a lot of conviction in the thinking that marriage could be successful if the partners see less of each other. The day time separation of the partners when they go to work may not be enough. Ideally, if the husband goes away even for short periods would tend to keep the togetherness of marriage alive, fresh and full of desire. To relieve the boredom of seeing each other all the time, it would be so much better if both husband and wife, accept each other's need to meet their friends at the pub or local and at coffee meetings. What is the use of having a dinner date when husband and wife do not exchange a word and look utterly miserable and bored in each other's company unlike the courting days when even inane conversation was so animated and holding hands across the table embarrassed the serving waiter.

Unlike western countries where divorce is a significant part of marriage, and even the practical but unsavoury prenuptial agreement is thought of prior to tying the

knot, in India marriage is reckoned to be an unbreakable bond in life. It can be safely said that nearly 80 % of marriages in urban India and 99% in rural are arranged and there is very little of pre- marriage dating or courting and the man may be said to be literally purchasing the womb. Both the boy and the girl are usually in their teens and have first look at each other when the parents are negotiating the alliance which, amongst business houses, is a way to cement commercial ties. Parents show extreme apprehension if the girl is not settled in marriage before 20. Recently a statistical survey in the state in which I live revealed to my horror that that 40% of brides in urban areas and 52% in agricultural communities were married before the legal age of 18.

Early pregnancy is one of the most depressing cause of the ballooning population which is now estimated at 1100 + million with all its gargantuan problems of feeding, educating, finding employment and providing medical care for the people. But there is hope. More and more female education and empowerment are slowly changing the scenario and young college going boys and girls are increasingly dating and possibly making their personal choice and with it there will surely follow the need to limit families for a better standard of living.

The downside of arranged marriages where couples have had no opportunity to size up what they are going to get was demonstrated in a recent case in India where the husband horrified his young wife in the bridal chamber on the first night by removing his wig and placing his

dentures on the table next to the bed. He looked much older than 24 and the terrified wife fled to her parents' home. Later it transpired that the wedding ornaments were also fake.

An off shoot of this are child marriages, particularly in Rajasthan, which are legally prohibited as the minimum marriage age is 18 when, to seal business ties, tiny tots are married in elaborate ceremonies and then live apart and stay with their parents, until they reach the age of puberty. This is one more instance where the law looks the other way which is nothing to be astonished at because in India laws abound for nearly every conceivable behaviour in life but the implementation is dismally poor.

In India, chastity is the most important requirement and it is presumed it is intact at the time of marriage. The man, no matter what a philanderer he has been, demands a virgin as a matter of right. Discussion of sex at home is taboo and swept under the carpet with absence of teaching at school in a nation which cries out for transparency and awareness of practice of birth control.

Until female empowerment with better education and community tolerance becomes widespread, a woman is supposed to stick to her husband and make the marriage work even though he may be a bounder prone to wild rages, battering, drinking and even unconcealed infidelity. In the mind of the wife he is really the lord and master who can do no wrong. In the Gujarati language he is referred to in common parlance as *dhani* which literally means owner or proprietor.

She may live in a state of acute unhappiness but she has nowhere to go. In case the woman abandons her marital home, she invites social ignominy and her parents may give her temporary shelter but at the same time some of them would go on dinning into her ears to return to her marital bed even though they know that they are condemning their own daughter to live the rest of her life in hell. They are also motivated by the idle patter of nosey neighbours along with Indian society which looks down unkindly on a divorcee or one who has left her married home. It is next to impossible for a divorcee to find a husband and remarry. It is such a pathetic drag on her life that there is no space or hope of longevity for her.

There is not the least doubt that a successful long lasting marriage full of compassion, companionship, tolerance and without acrimony will be a prime candidate for longevity as it will be free from stress which is mentally quite disturbing. In our fast moving modern times this would indeed be a difficult achievement but married couples despite infrequent glitches must make marriages work and give them a good try. Marriages full of bitterness, incompatibility and mutual dislike have no truck with longevity and is a life full of misery. I can never get out of my mind the photograph of the state visit of a royal couple to a foreign country, who whilst facing their hosts, showed all their incompatibility and mutual dislike by looking sideways in opposite directions. What misery was portrayed on their faces but fortunately they were divorced later.

Chapter VI

**"Too much of anything is bad
but too much of whisky is rarely enough"**

Mark Twain

Alcohol Smoking and Longevity

People are drinking liquor more than ever. Drinking has become a mark of achievement that "you have arrived" and it is "the thing" to indulge in to be upwardly mobile. More and more young people, particularly ladies, are getting used to heavy drinking. Women drinking at a public bar unknowingly have their drinks spiked by strangers and end up sexually outraged. They are abandoned dazed in a traumatic state in a strange decrepit place to rue the night out which has turned into a horror. One in three raped women in UK, when reporting rape, admitted to excessive drinking before the alleged offence, and many of them were so dazed, under the influence of heavy drinking, that they pleaded they were not even

sure they had been raped, which has resulted in barely 6% conviction. Alcohol is becoming a major contributory factor in rape of women.

Many ladies are known to go to bed mildly drunk every night. It is not the gin and tonic or whisky which draws them but it is the well stocked wine which is the favourite and the nightly routine. At a ladies dinner evening out, while some sensibly interrupt their booze with a non-alcoholic glass others carry on with their attack on the bottle as if wasting is a sin. It is not unusual to go through a bottle before the first course announces its presence. There can not be any celebration for a special event without wine being drunk in good quantities. They are not binge drinkers walking the pavements boisterously and singing happily as men do.

What should be a reasonable quantity? Medical advice is that women should not drink more than two to three units daily (about 8 units a bottle) or maximum 14 a week whilst men because they are muscularly bigger can go up to 4 a day and 21 in a week.

The French are great wine drinkers but strangely enough you don't find them drunk in the streets. The Germans and beer are inseparable and they generally drink in huge quantities. Their Munich beer fest is a delight to visit and participate where beer is served in mugs as large as the thigh. Austrians and the people of most central European countries are generally great beer drinkers.

The Russians mystical attachment to vodka has increased with visible presence in the streets of inebriated Russians. Despite life expectancy of 60, alcoholism amongst men is the most serious problem after heart disease and cancer. Alcoholism's annual death toll is 40,000 to 50,000 in a country facing a serious demographic problem with the population predicted to decline by 30% to 100 million by the middle of this century. The President of Russia is personally involved in curbing the Russians love for vodka in particular.

This addiction has led to embarrassing situation and the well known incident which comes to mind is the head of the Russian state, lying in a highly inebriated condition in the airliner, which brought him on a state visit to a European country. He was unable to emerge to be received by the representatives of the host state, who were left to cool their heels. The explanation given was of course that the visiting head was unwell and this high profile snafu was kept under wraps. The same head of state on another state visit broke ranks at a solemn function and suddenly snatched the conductor's baton and started conducting the band much to the amusement of the assembled gathering and he was completely oblivious to the embarrassment caused to his hosts. Not to be outdone, on another state occasion to Washington, he was accommodated as a state guest in Blair House, stone's throw from White House, and he was so inebriated that he was found wandering in Pennsylvania Avenue, in the dead of night allegedly in his

under pants, searching for a taxi and, when confronted by the alarmed secret service, he said he wanted a pizza!

The present trend is to liberalise drinking by legislation to liberate people from restrictions and appeal to their maturity to curtail heavy drinking. In UK, all pubs and drinking establishments serving liquor, which included beer, used to close by law officially at 11 pm. This was considered to be the cause of binge drinking with drinkers, loading themselves before closing time, and then pouring into the streets in drunk and disorderly state creating nuisance and inflicting a sense of social insecurity with a high potential for crime. I have been a witness to rowdy behaviour of frightening proportions of highly inebriated men on Saturday nights in the streets and subways after football matches.

Weight loss seekers must know that drink is calorie rich. A normal glass of wine taken daily, which is not harmful but on the contrary good for health, contains about 85 calories. A pint of beer will toss you for 190 calories and a bottle can mean 400. Whisky soda, and rum and coke will each set you back by 145 calories. Since hardly any one is satisfied with one glass and to be normally correct in the social ladder you have to let the evening roll, a repeat becomes a must which may not be the end. Multiply the intake by 2 and 3 and see what a disastrous quantity of calories have been added for the day which, unlike food, cannot be absorbed by any form of exercise or physical exertion. It is just an addition to your food bank with no quick facility for shedding.

This is not all and the worst is to come. Alcohol is the best appetite stimulant. It is said the aperitif was specially designed to create hunger but alcohol is the worst. Add chicken *tikka, kababs,* sausages which are easy prey to satiate your hunger. Is it realised what a destructive combination alcohol and food are at slimming efforts? Where and when are you going to get rid of the loads of calories added by this combination?

Apart from the dreaded weight gain there are the unpleasant side effects of excessive drinking which shows up in an abnormally flushed look, skin dehydration and disappearance of youthful glow, drowsiness, loss of libido, slobbering, hangover with headache and disorderly behaviour at home and in public. Continued heavy drinking could raise the deadly spectre of liver cihrossis which could be fatal.

I knew a friend who was a compulsive drinker of gin in his waking hours. He carried a flask wherever he went, and drank from it neat or slightly diluted with water, if the latter was easily available. The worst thing that could have happened to him was that he drank without lining his stomach with food, even in small quantities, until he developed cihrossis of the liver and died peacefully. He was a jolly, friendly type, who could have adorned his life and enriched that of his family, but no amount of compassionate remonstrance and pleading by family and friends to wean him away had any effect. Hundreds of thousands are similarly cutting short their lives dying in middle age through alcoholism suffering from liver disease

and otherwise face infertility, dementia, osteoporosis and even some types of cancer particularly amongst women

A glass of red wine at lunch and dinner is healthy and so is a peg of whisky which acts as a stimulant for the heart and the nervous system. I drink beer occasionally and Scotch and soda rarely. My favourite drink is a glass of wine sometimes with dinner. Moderation in drinking is the buzzword. Excess will spell disaster. I cannot subscribe to Mark Twain's aphorism "Too much of anything is bad but too much of whisky is rarely enough." Moderate drinking is also a great comforter and promotes a certain benign mental attitude. Don't we drink when we are happy and equally when we are sad (how often we have heard the expression "drowning my sorrows").

James I (1603-25) detested the "loathsome" habit of smoking but he did not mind encouraging it for his tax revenues. The spread of cigarette smoking could have originated from soldiers returning from the Crimean War acquiring the habit by watching Ottoman Turkish soldiers smoking.

There is so much said and written about smoking that there is very little one can add to its effects on health and longevity. Reduced lung capacity in extreme cases leading to such breathing problems that it is difficult to walk from one end of bedroom to another without the help of an oxygen bottle, loss of appetite and libido, foul breath, stained teeth, unhealthy pallor, constant coughing and never to be forgotten the high incidence of cancer are

some of the disastrous consequences. A recent research concluded that even one cigarette a day was harmful.

But smokers have a do or die attitude, and cigarette companies have never had it so good as now in sales and profitability. Nothing deters a committed habituated smoker from having his fag. Even the tell tale signs of impending disaster such as continuous coughing, hoarseness, dark sputum etc. are all brushed aside and ignored. Most smokers suffer from an element of cowardice refusing to submit to medical advice to undergo checks for fear of being confronted with dark news.

Smoking has now become the modern scourge of mankind. Nicotine addiction is worse than being high on cocaine. The number of people dying or incapacitated annually by smoking and smoke related diseases far outweigh the death toll from Katrina, Rita, tsunamis and hurricanes , typhoons, earthquakes and other devastating natural calamities which, from time to time, have left a trail of destruction and death.

It is estimated, that in India 2400 people die every day (876,000 per year) from tobacco related diseases which include the widespread nefarious habit of chewing tobacco in some form or the other. In USA nearly 400,000 are dying from smoking and smoke related diseases. Passive smoking affects nearly 300,000 children who develop low resistance to pneumonia, coughs, wheezing, asthma and other lung affected ailments. It is estimated that 10 million people will die annually from tobacco related illnesses by the year 2030. According to the World Bank

by that year tobacco will be the single biggest cause of death. What a disastrous and unnecessary short shrift to natural longevity. It is incomprehensible what leads mankind to knowingly fall prey to this scourge.

Studies in USA indicate that cigarette smokers are 70% more at risk from premature death than non-smokers. No amount of clamping on marketing and sales nor projecting its harmful effects in the most dramatic and explicit manner on the wrappers showing what would happen to the innards due to smoking nor imposing a ban on restaurants and enclosed public places, where people congregate, has had any measurable effect on reducing the number of smokers. To them it is "desire pursues like fell and cruel hounds" (Twelfth Night, Shakespeare).

Nevertheless, smoking is getting tougher by the day in many countries of the world. Prodigious efforts are being made by legislation and voluntary action to reduce smoking. It appears that, at the most, this has only resulted in arresting further increase although it is claimed that about 1.30 million Americans, particularly teenagers, stop smoking every year. Nobody has any idea of how many freshers take to smoking and become habituated.

Today Bhutan, the small Himalayan kingdom (pop.800,000), is the only country in the world which has imposed a total ban on smoking. Italy, Norway, Spain, Belgium, Northern Ireland and Scotland have banned smoking in all public places including restaurants, bars etc. In USA, California and New York have imposed similar bans. In France, smoking is banned in all public

places which includes all the captivating smoky cafes like Café de Flor, Café aux Deux Maggots on the left bank made famous by existentialists. Britain has already banned or is planning to prohibit smoking in areas where people gather which will include any enclosed public place, bus shelters, train platforms, big playgrounds to protect more people from being exposed to passive smoking. Already tube trains, restaurants, pubs are free of smokers.

Dissenters claim that this is a disproportionate response because there is no scientific evidence that passive smoking is harmful. In many restaurants, it is normal to segregate smoking and non-smoking areas, but the efficacy of this measure is doubtful, unless smokers are placed in a special enclosed area.

Some countries promote smoking for economic reasons. For cigar lovers Cuba is the obvious choice, with guided tours of establishments where cigars are rolled. Estonia also offers cigar tours. Spain and Portugal are still friendly. In China, Russia and Japan unrestricted smoking is permitted. In India restrictions are applied in public transport and closed areas such as cinema halls, theatres etc

Smoking and excessive and binge drinking are the sworn enemies of good health and a great deterrent to longevity. They debase a person's life and give no pleasure to people around him. To kick the habit is understandably difficult but if long healthy life is desired there can not be any compromise in getting rid of smoking altogether

and restricting drinking to reasonably socially acceptable levels.

A word of caution about the down side of giving up smoking is the gain in weight and possibly developing type 2 diabetes but this should not deter people from kicking the habit because it is a far better alternative than lung cancer and other health problems. Weight gain could be easily controlled by proper exercise regime and strict check on intake of food but you can not cure cancer of the lungs.

Epilogue

This century will be momentous if new researches for extending longevity are successful. In the light of scientific developments taking place to extend life span, my reaching 90 will be considered prosaic not worth commending except that this has been in the tropics particularly in the harsh environment of a country known for appalling hygiene, sanitation, medical facilities and the ever present soul destroying spectre of grinding poverty and under nourishment of nearly 400 millions in whose midst I have lived my life.

All over the world scientists, in well funded and endowed laboratories and research centres, are relentlessly pursuing the goal of identifying what causes diseases which afflict mankind limiting life span and are attempting to find remedies to conquer them. Will the child born today live long enough and cross a century and beyond even up to 150 with a healthy life style if not struck down unfortunately by accidents, Tsunamis or wars waged by

politicians? Will the planet be awash with handsome faces drinking eternally from the fountain of youth?

The conquest of ageing with mental alacrity for those in their 60s and 70s is not far away with advances in biology, biotechnology, genetics and stem cell researches which will identify and repair damages affecting vital organs causing life threatening illnesses leading to untimely death. If ongoing researches discover how organs age (senescence) there is hope even for some sort of immortality.

Scientists are continuing to figure out how some people live up to 100 enjoying good health. This seems to be a contradiction because at 100 how can one have good health and physical energy to enjoy life and not lie on a nursing home bed. Nevertheless whilst researchers accept that genetic factors do play a part in longevity, most importantly it is good life style, healthy diet and refreshing environment which are very important for longevity. Scientists researching for achieving longevity must necessarily do so without a hospital bed so that centenarians who number 450,000 today in western developed countries and likely to reach an estimated one million by 2030 lead a healthy meaningful life.

What will it all look like then with a significant proportion of people you meet are above 100? Will life on the planet, which even now is bursting with 6 billion, be sustainable for food, housing, conservancy, medical services, education and social intercourse? We cannot manage 6 billions today with widespread hunger and present rate of mortality but if people were to live longer

will Malthus wake up from his slumber and remind mankind of his law? How will we tackle requirement of adequate supplies of food with land eroding without climate control? In the present social fabric what will be the new retirement age? These questions can only be ignored with peril and need to be addressed.

Also is mankind going to pay heed to the alarming signals of earth warming which continues unabated despite all the awareness and agreement reached of the need to take corrective steps at the recently concluded Copenhagen summit? It is not only the destruction of virgin forests which will have a big effect on earth warming but the unchecked heat emission leading to the inexorable reduction in the arctic snow cap. Already the polar bear, the symbol of earth warming, is swimming and swimming to reach a reasonable sheet of ice to raise her cubs and look for the life sustaining snout of seals for food for her family, but this appears to be more and more distant.

On a personal level what is in store for me? How many more days to go (it would be absurd to talk of years no matter how positive I am). Naturally bizarre thoughts float in my mind. Where will I be going? If I were to quote the late Art Buchwald I shouldn't think this way without explaining what business I have to be here in the first instance.

Am I frightened? No. What is there to be frightened of or be glad about? 90 years and possibly more with reasonable affluence and very enviable health is immense

provenance which God the Almighty has provided to me. As I prepare to face the inevitable I take immense pleasure that I have gone through my life causing least harm to any one except for human frailties which sometimes may have made me transgress my self- imposed limits of behaviour.

I have spent my adult life witnessing widespread historical convulsions. I have been witness to the Second World War resulting in the deaths of 25 millions, the birth of Stalinism, the Chinese, Russian and Cuban revolutions, Pearl Harbour, the Holocaust, the Berlin Wall and its destruction later, the wars in North Korea and Viet Nam, the dropping of the atom bombs on Japan, the Independence of India and African countries, the resurgence of China and India as the future economic power houses and 65 years of peace descending on the planet without a major world war. What more does one want to grip attention?

There are neither devils awaiting me with lethal lances nor virgins to take me in their arms. There will be no roasting in oil or walking in a garden brimful with roses. Nor are my departed beloved parents, my brothers, my sister and my dearest wife waiting to welcome me in their folds. Neither Orion will halt to unsheathe his sword to protect me nor Pegasus offer to show me the delights of God's domain. There is nothing but nothingness facing me.

I have written so much about the need to believe in God and religion that the reader will think I am talking

as if I hate atheists. No, this is too simplistic a view. Belief in God and faith in one's religion without all its miracles, myths and fables are vehicles which propel one through life by detachment from stark materialism. For a thoughtful individual Heaven and Hell are just apparitions and not an engine driving one to be good or bad through life.

I am relaxed and very calm. I have had a full enjoyable life largely free from distress and calamities except one when I suddenly lost my wife in tragic circumstances 52 years ago after 10 years of a very happy marriage. This was a lightning bolt leaving me with two daughters who were 8 and 3 years of age. I was devastated with the loss and overwhelmed with new responsibility. Imagine a single man facing the reality of looking after two tiny tots and taking them through education, grooming, puberty, initiation into religion, protecting them and marrying them to men of their choice who have been splendid husbands and fathers.

Will I have any regrets to leave my footprints for ever and just float away into oblivion? Yes, of course. I am reasonably well off but abandoning all the glitter is the least regret. I started life with practically nothing and this is how I will go unshackled and unburdened with a sneaking thought that all that is left behind is self-made.

But surely I would miss my family? Indeed if I had the consciousness to miss them. I would hate to leave my two charming daughters who came under my sole care when they were 8 and 3 years of age and are now 61 and 56. Their devotion, care, compassion and attachment

have brought me great peace and contentment. They have grown into classy, elegant, educated ladies who would be ornaments in any family. Both are amateur artists and one of them is a successful professional landscape architect. Out of three grandchildren one is working as a banker in London, the second is in the media profession and the youngest in his teens is at school settled in London with his parents. They have been the joys of my life ever since the first was born in 1982.

Finally, despite all the shortcomings and difficult conditions of life I will truly and sincerely cannot forget my country India. I was born and educated here, made a satisfactory career, raised a family, and had enough money to live free from want. Whatever I am today I owe everything to India and the opportunities it created for me to be successful.

But I remain overwhelmed by the condition of millions of the poor for whose uplift I regret I have been unable to do anything. This state of poverty is principally due to appalling governance with governments on the brink of bankruptcy and the endemic corrupt politicians and bureaucracy. The only pall on my life is the overwhelming guilt of enjoying a life style way above the millions who are hungry and without shelter. I sincerely hope and pray that future economic development is more inclusive leading to vast improvement in their lives in the next 10-15 years and my daughters and grand children see their co-nationals enjoying a better life.

India is a beautiful fascinating country. Its 5000 year old culture, diversity of people, religions and faiths epitomised with 17 major languages, its mighty rivers meandering through the length and breadth of the country, its mountains which are the highest in the world peaking with snow, its unparallel fauna and flora, its huge variety of cuisine, its argumentative and noisy people and querulous parliamentarians, its beautiful women make India a truly captivating country. It is said that the diversity in India is so compelling that after every 400 miles you see a different India in dressage, cuisine, habits, religious beliefs, traditions and language.

I have never felt like leaving India and settling abroad as some of my friends are itching to do. Whenever I have gone abroad after a short time India has irresistibly drawn me back home with a powerful magnet. I am reminded of a resident of Timbuktu (part of west African Mali in the Sahara desert) living in Paris but yearning for his city and missing the violent sand storms, dry arid climate and even the braying of donkeys.

As Somerset Maugham said "Dying is a very dull, dreary affair. And my advice to you is to have nothing whatever to do with it". When my time comes I pray it will not be with help of physicians with the body plastered with tubes and drips and transfusions. "The goal of all life is death" (Sigmund Freud) and we have to pray that when it comes it will be peaceful.

About the Author
Minoo Vazifdar

The author, who lives in Mumbai (Bombay), is an Indian in his 92nd year. He is a Master in Economics and has attended the high management course at Henley-on Thames, UK. The French Government in 1988 conferred on him the title of Chevalier de L'Ordre National du Merite.

He brings to bear in his writing unrivalled experience of life having been an interested spectator since age 20 of the great upheavals caused by the Second World War and the convulsions which followed with the horrific Russian and Chinese revolutions, the drop of the atom bomb and the Independence granted to India which was followed by independence of several countries in Africa, south-east Asia and other parts of the world. All this changed the face of the planet and the way people lived and their beliefs.

His thoughts and perceptions are not rigid. He is deeply religious but tolerant of those who are not. He has looked at the world as if people are walking on the bridge of mortality without camping engaged in petty quarrels, greed, excesses, selfishness and generally in an unfulfilled and unhappy life. Without claiming to be a student of human frailties he has evolved by personal experience what should be the way to longevity, and not an early hospital bed, by following certain disciplines which are not draconian but simple to follow.

He emphasises that reaching 60/65 is not the end of life but the beginning of the new 80s. There is a universal urge amongst mankind to live as long as possible and it is here that he is trying to make a practical contribution without frills in his book

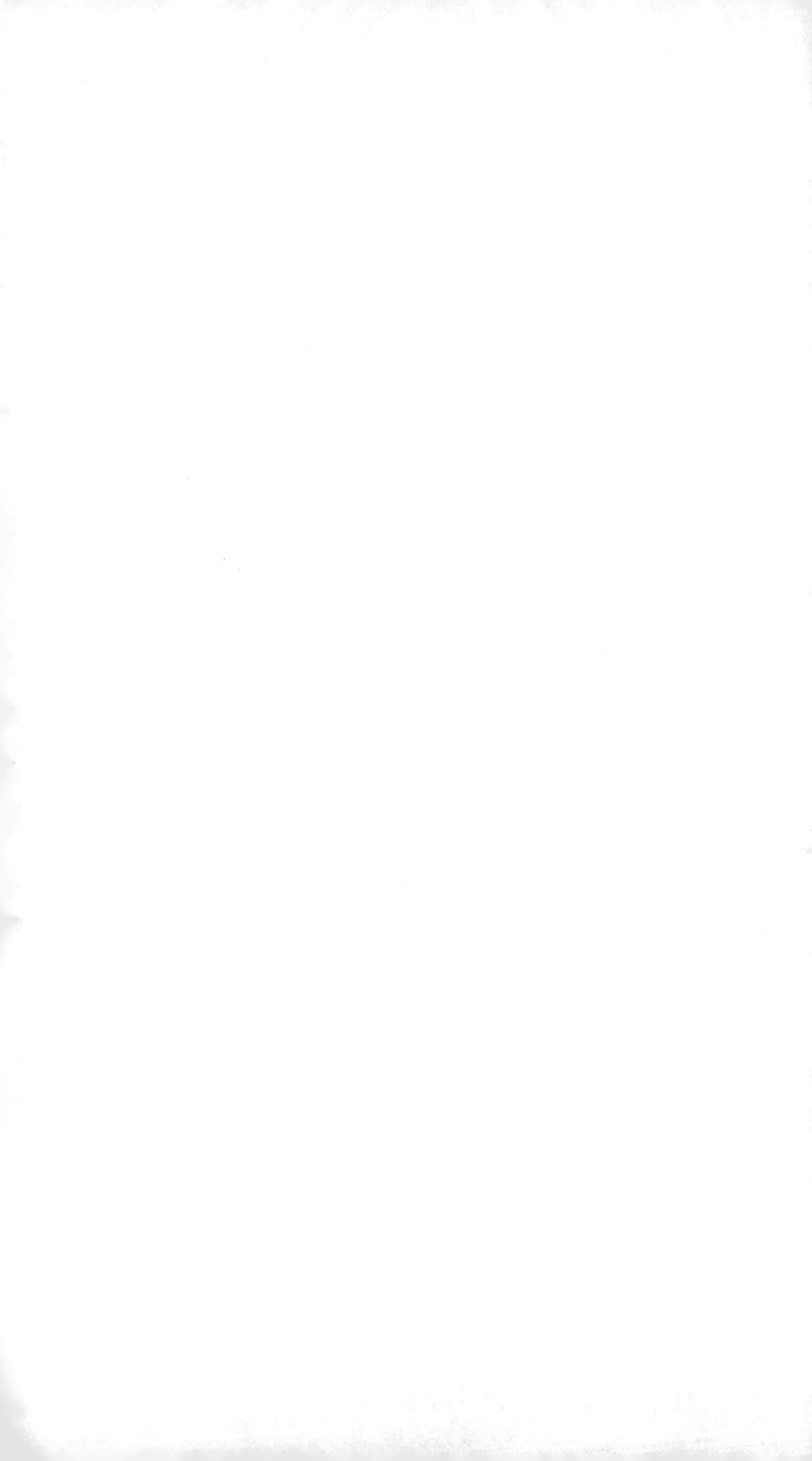

www.ingramcontent.com/pod-product-compliance
Lightning Source LLC
Chambersburg PA
CBHW020440290526
45785CB00002B/939

I0449599